Psychiatric Mental Health Nursing Case Studies

Real-World Scenarios and Evidence-Based Clinical Practice

Alma Aradia Peterson

This publication is intended for educational use by licensed healthcare professionals, nursing students, and healthcare educators. It should not be used as a substitute for proper clinical training, supervision, or continuing education requirements.

ISBN: 978-1-7641942-5-9

Isohan Publishing

Table of Contents

Chapter 1: Introduction to Case-Based Learning in Psychiatric Nursing 1

Chapter 2: Essential Assessment Skills and Tools 6

Chapter 3: Therapeutic Communication and Relationship Building 14

Chapter 4: Legal and Ethical Foundations 22

Chapter 5: Care Planning Frameworks 32

Chapter 6: Inpatient Psychiatric Unit Cases.................................44

Chapter 7: Emergency Department Psychiatric Emergencies 57

Chapter 8: Outpatient and Community Mental Health.................................68

Chapter 9: Specialized Populations and Settings.................................80

Chapter 10: Technology-Enhanced Psychiatric Care 94

Chapter 11: Emerging Mental Health Challenges 107

Chapter 12: Complex Multi-System Cases.................................123

Chapter 13: Crisis Intervention and Disaster Response 140

Chapter 14: Quality Improvement and Evidence-Based Practice 154

Chapter 15: Professional Development and Self-Care 169

References 184

Chapter 1: Introduction to Case-Based Learning in Psychiatric Nursing

The human mind presents one of nursing's most complex challenges. Unlike a broken bone that shows clearly on an X-ray or a wound that can be measured and photographed, mental health conditions require a different kind of assessment—one that relies on observation, conversation, and clinical reasoning. This is where case-based learning becomes not just helpful, but essential for developing competent psychiatric nurses.

You are about to enter a learning experience that mirrors real clinical practice. Instead of memorizing lists of symptoms or theoretical frameworks in isolation, you'll work through actual patient scenarios that unfold just as they do in hospitals, clinics, and community settings. Each case builds your clinical reasoning skills while teaching you to think like an experienced psychiatric nurse.

Learning Objectives Framework

The American Association of Colleges of Nursing (AACN) Essentials 2021 provides the foundation for this textbook (1, 2). These ten domains guide everything from your first patient interaction to your development as a professional nurse. The domains most relevant to psychiatric nursing include:

Domain 1: Knowledge for Nursing Practice focuses on understanding mental health across the lifespan. You'll learn to recognize normal psychological development and identify deviations that signal mental health concerns.

Domain 3: Population Health addresses the social determinants that affect mental health. Poverty, discrimination, trauma, and social isolation all play roles in psychiatric conditions. Through case studies, you'll see how these factors influence patient care and recovery.

Domain 6: Interprofessional Partnerships becomes critical in psychiatric settings where social workers, psychiatrists, therapists, and peer support specialists work together. Each case study includes interprofessional elements to prepare you for collaborative practice.

Domain 9: Professionalism addresses the ethical challenges unique to psychiatric nursing. Issues of autonomy, beneficence, and justice take on special meaning when patients may lack insight into their conditions or capacity to make decisions.

Domain 10: Personal, Professional, and Leadership Development recognizes that psychiatric nursing affects practitioners deeply. You'll learn self-awareness techniques and resilience strategies to maintain your own mental health while caring for others.

Clinical Reasoning Models

Two proven frameworks guide your thinking through complex psychiatric cases. **Tanner's Clinical Judgment Model** consists of four phases: noticing, interpreting, responding, and reflecting (3). This model helps you develop pattern recognition skills that experienced nurses use intuitively.

The **Outcome-Present State-Test (OPT) Model** provides a systematic approach to care planning. You identify desired outcomes, assess the current situation, and determine what tests or interventions will move the patient toward recovery goals. Both models integrate throughout this textbook's case studies.

Progressive Complexity Approach

This textbook follows evidence-based principles of adult learning. Simple cases appear first, allowing you to practice basic skills before tackling complex scenarios (4). Each chapter builds on previous knowledge while introducing new concepts.

Green Level Cases focus on single diagnoses with clear presentations. A patient with major depression and obvious symptoms provides a straightforward learning experience.

Yellow Level Cases involve multiple factors or comorbid conditions. A patient with bipolar disorder who also has diabetes requires more complex thinking about medication interactions and self-care abilities.

Red Level Cases present ethical dilemmas, cultural complexities, or multiple systems involvement. A homeless veteran with PTSD, substance use disorder, and legal problems challenges you to coordinate care across multiple agencies while advocating for patient needs.

Case Study 1.1: Learning Through Experience

Maria Santos, a 28-year-old teacher, arrives at the emergency department after her husband found her crying uncontrollably in their bedroom. She tells the triage nurse, "I can't stop thinking about hurting myself. I'm scared of what I might do."

Your Initial Response: What do you notice first about Maria's presentation? The obvious answer might be her suicidal ideation, but experienced nurses notice more. Her ability to recognize dangerous thoughts and seek help demonstrates insight and protective factors.

Her husband's involvement suggests social support. These observations become part of your clinical reasoning process.

Unfolding Scenario: As you gather more information, you learn Maria stopped taking her antidepressant medication two weeks ago because she "felt better." She's been sleeping only 2-3 hours nightly and hasn't eaten in two days. Her teaching job, which she usually loves, has become overwhelming.

This case teaches medication adherence, early warning signs of depression relapse, and the importance of patient education. You'll follow Maria through emergency assessment, safety planning, and coordination with outpatient providers.

Case Study 1.2: Cultural Considerations in Assessment

Ahmed Hassan, a 45-year-old engineer who immigrated from Lebanon five years ago, presents with his adult daughter for psychiatric evaluation. His daughter explains that her father has been "acting strange" for the past month—talking to himself, refusing to leave the house, and expressing fears that neighbors are watching him.

Cultural Competence Challenge: Your assessment must consider cultural factors that might influence Ahmed's presentation. In some cultures, spiritual experiences that might appear psychotic to Western practitioners are normal. Language barriers can complicate mental status examinations. Family dynamics around mental health vary significantly across cultures.

Progressive Learning: This case introduces cultural formulation concepts from the DSM-5-TR while teaching basic psychosis assessment skills. You'll learn to distinguish cultural practices from pathological symptoms while providing culturally responsive care.

Case Study 1.3: Technology Integration

Jennifer Park, a 34-year-old marketing executive, participates in telepsychiatry services due to her rural location. During a video session, she appears agitated and reports increasing anxiety since starting a new job. The connection keeps cutting out, making assessment challenging.

Technology Considerations: This case teaches telehealth assessment skills, including how to evaluate mental status through video platforms. You'll learn to adapt communication techniques for virtual encounters and understand the limitations of remote psychiatric care.

Modern Practice Reality: With telehealth becoming standard practice, especially after COVID-19, these skills are essential for contemporary psychiatric nursing practice.

Self-Assessment Tools

Before beginning each chapter, complete competency checklists that help identify your learning needs. These tools aren't tests—they're guides for focusing your study efforts. If you've never assessed suicide risk, spend extra time on those sections. If you've worked in medical-surgical nursing, you might already understand documentation requirements.

Pre-Learning Assessment Example:

- Can you identify the components of a mental status examination?
- Do you know the difference between hallucinations and delusions?
- Have you ever used a standardized depression screening tool?
- Are you familiar with psychiatric medications and their side effects?

Honest self-assessment guides your learning journey and helps you track progress as you develop expertise.

Technology Integration

Modern psychiatric nursing increasingly involves technology. Electronic health records capture assessment data differently than paper charts. Patients use smartphone apps to track moods and medication adherence. Nurses participate in telehealth encounters and monitor patients through remote sensors.

Virtual Reality Applications: Some clinical sites now use VR for exposure therapy with PTSD patients or social skills training for patients with autism spectrum disorders. Understanding these technologies prepares you for evolving practice environments.

Digital Resources: Each chapter includes QR codes linking to video demonstrations, interactive simulations, and current research articles. These supplements expand your learning beyond traditional textbook formats.

Building Your Clinical Reasoning Foundation

As you work through cases, pay attention to your thinking process. Expert nurses don't just know facts—they recognize patterns, anticipate complications, and intervene before problems escalate. This intuitive knowledge develops through repeated exposure to patient situations.

Document your reasoning as you work through cases. Write down your initial impressions, list questions that arise, and note how additional information changes your thinking. This reflection process accelerates your development from novice to competent practitioner.

The journey ahead challenges you to think differently about nursing care. Medical-surgical patients often present with clear-cut problems requiring procedural interventions. Psychiatric patients present with complex human experiences requiring therapeutic relationships, cultural sensitivity, and ethical reasoning.

Key Learning Points

Remember these essential principles as you begin:

- Every patient interaction offers learning opportunities
- Cultural competence requires ongoing self-reflection and education
- Technology supports but never replaces therapeutic relationships
- Clinical reasoning develops through practice and reflection
- Self-care isn't selfish—it's necessary for effective patient care

Reflections on Professional Growth

The cases ahead will challenge your assumptions about mental illness, recovery, and human resilience. Patients will surprise you with their strength, frustrate you with their choices, and teach you about courage in ways you never expected. This is the beginning of a professional journey that transforms not just your nursing practice, but your understanding of what it means to be human.

Your success in psychiatric nursing depends less on memorizing diagnostic criteria and more on developing genuine compassion for people experiencing their most difficult moments. The technical skills matter, but the therapeutic relationship you build with patients often determines treatment outcomes. This textbook prepares you for both aspects of practice.

Chapter 2: Essential Assessment Skills and Tools

Walking into a patient's room for the first time requires a particular kind of awareness. You observe not just what the patient says, but how they say it. You notice posture, eye contact, grooming, and countless other details that inform your clinical picture. In psychiatric nursing, assessment never stops—it continues throughout every interaction.

The mental status examination serves as your primary assessment tool, but it's more than a checklist to complete. It's a systematic way of organizing observations about a person's psychological functioning at a specific point in time. Think of it as taking vital signs of the mind.

Mental Status Examination Components

Appearance provides your first clinical data. Does the patient appear their stated age? Are they dressed appropriately for the season and setting? Grooming offers clues about functional capacity and self-care abilities. A disheveled appearance might indicate depression, cognitive impairment, or substance use—but it could also reflect homelessness or cultural differences in dress.

Behavior encompasses both obvious actions and subtle movements. Restlessness might suggest anxiety, medication side effects, or akathisia from antipsychotic medications. Repetitive behaviors could indicate obsessive-compulsive disorder or autism spectrum conditions. Note whether the patient makes eye contact, follows social cues, and responds appropriately to your presence.

Speech assessment goes beyond content to include rate, volume, and rhythm. Pressured speech often accompanies mania, while monotone delivery might suggest depression or schizophrenia. Listen for accent, language fluency, and vocabulary level—these factors affect how you structure your assessment questions.

Mood represents the patient's subjective emotional state—what they tell you they're feeling. **Affect** describes your objective observation of their emotional expression. A patient might report feeling "fine" while appearing tearful and anxious. This incongruence between mood and affect provides important clinical information.

Thought Process evaluation examines how ideas connect and flow. Logical, goal-directed thinking is normal. Flight of ideas, where thoughts jump rapidly between topics, suggests mania. Circumstantial thinking includes excessive detail but eventually reaches the point. Tangential thinking never returns to the original topic.

Thought Content focuses on what the patient thinks about. Delusions are fixed false beliefs that resist logical argument. Obsessions are persistent, intrusive thoughts that cause distress. Suicidal or homicidal ideation requires immediate assessment of intent, plan, and means.

Perceptual Disturbances include hallucinations in any sensory modality. Auditory hallucinations are most common in psychiatric conditions. Visual hallucinations might suggest medical causes like delirium or substance intoxication. Always ask about command hallucinations that instruct patients to harm themselves or others.

Cognitive Function testing includes orientation, attention, memory, and executive functioning. Simple questions like "What year is it?" assess orientation. Attention can be tested by having patients spell "world" backwards or count backwards from 100 by sevens. Memory testing should include both recent and remote recall.

Insight refers to the patient's understanding of their condition. Poor insight doesn't mean low intelligence—many highly educated people lack awareness of their mental illness during acute episodes. Insight often improves with treatment and can be a marker of recovery.

Judgment assessment examines decision-making capacity. Ask hypothetical questions like "What would you do if you found a stamped, addressed envelope on the sidewalk?" or "What would you do if you smelled smoke in a movie theater?" Poor judgment might indicate cognitive impairment, impulsivity, or acute psychiatric symptoms.

Case Study 2.1: Comprehensive Mental Status Assessment

Robert Chen, a 42-year-old accountant, presents to the emergency department after his supervisor called 911 when Robert began shouting about "government surveillance through the computer monitors" at work.

Appearance: Robert appears disheveled despite wearing a business suit. His hair is uncombed, he has food stains on his shirt, and he smells of body odor suggesting poor hygiene for several days.

Behavior: He sits rigidly in the chair, frequently glancing at the ceiling corners where he believes cameras are hidden. He startles when staff members enter the room and demands to see their identification badges.

Speech: His speech is rapid and loud. He uses technical jargon and speaks in long, complex sentences that are difficult to follow. His voice has an urgent, pressured quality.

Mood and Affect: Robert reports feeling "alert and necessary for national security." His affect appears anxious and suspicious, with periods of irritability when questioned about his beliefs.

Thought Process: His thinking shows flight of ideas, jumping from computer surveillance to international conspiracies to his college roommate who "might be involved." Connections between topics are loose and hard to follow.

Thought Content: He expresses grandiose delusions about being selected for a special government mission. He believes his work computer monitors his thoughts and transmits them to federal agencies. No suicidal ideation is expressed, but he mentions "eliminating security threats" if necessary.

Perceptual Disturbances: Robert reports hearing voices through the ventilation system that give him "mission updates." He denies visual hallucinations but frequently looks around as if responding to sounds others don't hear.

Cognitive Function: He's oriented to person and place but believes the date is "classified information." His attention is poor due to distractibility. Recent memory appears intact, but he interprets neutral events as having special significance.

Insight and Judgment: Robert has no insight into having a mental illness. He believes others fail to understand the importance of his mission. His judgment is severely impaired—he stopped going home because he fears his apartment is "compromised."

This assessment reveals acute psychosis requiring immediate intervention. The combination of paranoid delusions, command hallucinations, and impaired judgment creates significant safety concerns for Robert and potentially others.

Standardized Assessment Tools

While clinical observation provides rich qualitative data, standardized tools offer quantifiable measures for tracking treatment progress and ensuring consistent assessment across different clinicians.

Columbia Suicide Severity Rating Scale

The C-SSRS provides a systematic approach to suicide risk assessment (5, 6). This tool distinguishes between passive death wishes and active suicidal plans with specific methods and timelines. The scale addresses six categories of suicidal ideation and four types of suicidal behavior.

Ideation Categories:

1. Wish to be dead

2. Non-specific active suicidal thoughts

3. Active suicidal ideation with methods

4. Active suicidal ideation with intent

5. Active suicidal ideation with plan

6. Active suicidal ideation with plan and intent

Behavior Categories:

1. Preparatory acts

2. Aborted attempts

3. Interrupted attempts

4. Actual attempts

Case Study 2.2: Suicide Risk Assessment

Lisa Williams, a 19-year-old college freshman, presents to student health services reporting "feeling overwhelmed" since starting college six weeks ago. She appears tearful and states, "Sometimes I wonder if everyone would be better off without me."

C-SSRS Assessment Process:

Screening Questions: Lisa endorses wishing she were dead and having thoughts of killing herself. This positive screening requires full assessment.

Ideation Assessment: She reports thinking about suicide "a few times a week" but hasn't thought about specific methods. She denies intent, stating "I would never actually do it because of my family."

Behavior Assessment: Lisa denies any preparatory behaviors, aborted attempts, or actual suicide attempts. She has no history of self-harm behaviors.

Risk Factors: Recent major life transition, family history of depression (mother), academic stress, social isolation, and perfectionist personality traits.

Protective Factors: Strong family relationships, religious beliefs, fear of death, and future goals including graduate school.

Clinical Decision: Based on C-SSRS scoring, Lisa presents with low-moderate suicide risk. Outpatient treatment with close follow-up is appropriate, but she doesn't require psychiatric hospitalization.

This case demonstrates how standardized tools guide clinical decision-making while considering individual patient factors.

PHQ-9 and GAD-7 Administration

The Patient Health Questionnaire-9 measures depression severity, while the Generalized Anxiety Disorder-7 scale assesses anxiety symptoms (7, 8). Both tools take just minutes to complete and provide valuable baseline and outcome measures.

PHQ-9 Scoring:

- 0-4: Minimal depression
- 5-9: Mild depression
- 10-14: Moderate depression
- 15-19: Moderately severe depression
- 20-27: Severe depression

GAD-7 Scoring:

- 0-4: Minimal anxiety
- 5-9: Mild anxiety
- 10-14: Moderate anxiety
- 15-21: Severe anxiety

Montreal Cognitive Assessment

The MoCA provides a brief cognitive screening tool more sensitive than the Mini-Mental State Examination for detecting mild cognitive impairment (9, 10). The 30-point test assesses multiple cognitive domains including attention, executive function, memory, and visuospatial abilities.

Key Advantages:

- Detects mild cognitive changes

- Available in multiple languages

- Takes 10-15 minutes to administer

- Provides objective cognitive baseline

Case Study 2.3: Cognitive Assessment in Older Adults

Margaret O'Sullivan, an 78-year-old retired teacher, is brought to the clinic by her daughter who reports "Mom seems confused lately and forgets things she used to remember easily."

MoCA Administration Results:

- Visuospatial/Executive: 3/5 (difficulty with clock drawing and cube copy)

- Naming: 3/3 (correctly identified animals)

- Memory: 0/5 (recalled none of five words after delay)

- Attention: 4/6 (some difficulty with calculations and digit span)

- Language: 2/3 (struggled with sentence repetition)

- Abstraction: 1/2 (difficulty identifying similarities)

- Delayed Recall: 0/5 (no improvement with cueing)

- Orientation: 6/6 (fully oriented)

Total Score: 19/30 (adjusted to 20/30 with education correction)

This score suggests mild cognitive impairment requiring further evaluation. The pattern of deficits—particularly in memory and executive function—warrants neurological consultation and consideration of dementia screening.

Cultural Assessment Considerations

The DSM-5-TR Cultural Formulation Interview provides a structured approach to understanding how cultural factors influence mental health presentations (11, 12). This tool helps clinicians avoid misdiagnosis based on cultural misunderstandings.

Key Cultural Domains:

- Cultural identity and background

- Cultural conceptualizations of distress

- Psychosocial stressors and cultural features of vulnerability

- Cultural features of the relationship between patient and clinician

- Overall cultural assessment for diagnosis and care

Documentation Standards

Proper documentation protects patients, supports clinical decision-making, and meets regulatory requirements. The Joint Commission and Centers for Medicare & Medicaid Services have specific documentation standards for psychiatric care (13, 14).

Essential Documentation Elements:

- Date, time, and duration of assessment

- Patient identification and consent for treatment

- Chief complaint in patient's own words

- Mental status examination findings

- Risk assessment including suicide and violence potential

- Clinical formulation and differential diagnosis

- Treatment plan with specific, measurable goals

- Provider signature and credentials

Building Assessment Expertise

Assessment skills develop through practice and repetition. Each patient encounter offers opportunities to refine your observation abilities and clinical reasoning. Pay attention to subtle changes in presentation that might signal improvement or deterioration.

Practice mental status examinations with willing family members or fellow students. Notice how culture, age, education, and individual personality affect presentation. Learn to distinguish normal variations from pathological findings.

Document your assessments thoroughly and review them with experienced clinicians. Ask for feedback on your observations and clinical reasoning. Experienced nurses can teach you to notice patterns and warning signs that take years to develop independently.

Synthesis and Clinical Application

Effective psychiatric assessment combines systematic observation with standardized tools and cultural sensitivity. No single assessment method provides complete information—successful nurses integrate multiple data sources to develop accurate clinical pictures.

Technology will continue changing assessment practices. Smartphone apps now help patients track symptoms between appointments. Wearable devices monitor sleep patterns and activity levels. Artificial intelligence assists with diagnostic screening. Stay current with these developments while maintaining focus on therapeutic relationships that remain central to psychiatric nursing practice.

The skills you develop in assessment form the foundation for all other nursing interventions. Accurate assessment leads to appropriate diagnoses, effective treatment plans, and better patient outcomes. Master these fundamentals before moving to more complex clinical scenarios.

Key Principles to Remember:

- Assessment is ongoing, not a one-time event

- Standardized tools supplement but don't replace clinical judgment

- Cultural factors significantly influence mental health presentations

- Documentation must be thorough, accurate, and timely

- Safety assessment takes priority over all other considerations

- Practice improves both observation skills and efficiency

Your assessment expertise will determine your effectiveness as a psychiatric nurse. Patients trust you to understand their experiences accurately and respond appropriately to their needs. This responsibility requires continuous learning and professional development throughout your career.

Chapter 3: Therapeutic Communication and Relationship Building

The words you choose and how you say them can mean the difference between a patient who trusts you enough to share their darkest thoughts and one who remains silent behind a wall of fear and shame. In psychiatric nursing, communication isn't just about exchanging information—it's the primary therapeutic tool you have to help patients heal.

Therapeutic communication differs fundamentally from social conversation. While social interactions focus on mutual sharing and entertainment, therapeutic communication maintains a professional focus on patient needs and treatment goals. This doesn't mean being cold or distant—authentic warmth and empathy are essential—but your personal agenda never enters the conversation.

Foundation Skills for Therapeutic Relationships

Empathy forms the cornerstone of therapeutic communication. This means understanding and sharing your patient's emotional experience without becoming overwhelmed by it. You listen not just to words but to the pain, fear, hope, or confusion beneath them. When a patient says "I'm fine" while tears stream down their face, empathy helps you respond to their emotional reality rather than their words.

Genuineness requires you to be authentic in your interactions while maintaining professional boundaries. Patients can sense when you're being fake or going through the motions. They need to know you see them as a whole person, not just a diagnosis or problem to solve. This authenticity builds trust that encourages honest communication.

Positive regard means accepting patients without judgment, regardless of their behaviors, choices, or circumstances. This doesn't mean approving of everything they do—you can express concern about harmful behaviors while still communicating respect for their inherent worth as human beings.

Case Study 3.1: Building Rapport with a Resistant Adolescent

Tyler Jackson, a 16-year-old high school junior, was brought to the adolescent mental health unit by his parents after threatening to kill himself during a family argument. He sits with arms crossed, refusing to make eye contact, and responds to questions with single words or silence.

Initial Approach: Many nurses make the mistake of trying to rush past Tyler's resistance with direct questions about his suicidal thoughts. A more effective approach acknowledges his feelings about being there.

Nurse: "This probably isn't how you planned to spend your afternoon."

Tyler (looking up slightly): "You think?"

Nurse: "I'm guessing you're pretty angry about being here."

Tyler: "Wouldn't you be?"

Building Connection: Notice how the nurse doesn't immediately jump into assessment questions. Instead, she validates Tyler's likely feelings and invites him to express them. This approach demonstrates respect for his autonomy and helps establish common ground.

Nurse: "Yeah, I probably would be. It sounds like things got pretty intense at home."

Tyler: "My parents freak out about everything. I said one thing and suddenly I'm here talking to you."

Progression: Tyler's response reveals more information about the situation while expressing his perspective. The nurse continues to validate his feelings while gently exploring the circumstances.

Nurse: "That must have been scary for them to hear. What did you say that worried them so much?"

Tyler: "I just said maybe they'd be happier if I wasn't around anymore. I didn't mean I was actually going to do anything."

Therapeutic Response: The nurse now has important clinical information about Tyler's suicidal ideation while maintaining the therapeutic relationship. She can address safety concerns while continuing to show respect for his feelings and perspective.

This interaction demonstrates how therapeutic communication can overcome initial resistance by focusing on understanding rather than interrogation.

De-escalation Techniques

Aggressive or agitated patients require specialized communication approaches that prioritize safety while maintaining therapeutic relationships (15, 16). De-escalation involves verbal and non-verbal techniques designed to reduce tension and prevent violence.

Environmental Awareness: Position yourself between the patient and the exit. Maintain a safe distance—about arm's length—and avoid cornering the patient. Remove potential weapons like pens, scissors, or medical equipment from reach.

Non-verbal Communication: Keep your hands visible and open. Avoid sudden movements or gestures that might be perceived as threatening. Maintain a calm facial expression and moderate eye contact—too little seems dismissive, too much can feel confrontational.

Verbal Techniques: Speak slowly and calmly in a lower tone of voice. Use simple, clear language. Avoid arguing with delusions or trying to convince the patient they're wrong. Instead, focus on feelings and immediate concerns.

Case Study 3.2: Managing Aggressive Patient Interactions

David Martinez, a 35-year-old construction worker, presents to the emergency department intoxicated and agitated after a bar fight. He's pacing the room, clenching his fists, and shouting about "people trying to control" him.

Initial Assessment: David appears paranoid and hypervigilant. His speech is loud and rapid. He repeatedly asks about leaving and becomes more agitated when told he needs medical clearance first.

De-escalation Approach:

Nurse (standing near the door, hands visible): "David, I can see you're really upset about being here."

David: "You're damn right I'm upset! Nobody has the right to keep me here!"

Nurse: "That's a really frustrating feeling. Help me understand what's most concerning to you right now."

David: "I need to get out of here! People are after me and I'm trapped in this room!"

Validation and Redirection: The nurse acknowledges David's fears without agreeing with any paranoid content.

Nurse: "It sounds like you feel unsafe and trapped. I want to help you feel more comfortable. What would help you feel safer right now?"

David (pausing his pacing): "I just need to know I can leave when I want to."

Nurse: "I understand that feeling trapped makes this worse. The doctor needs to make sure you're not injured from the fight, and then we can talk about next steps. Can I get you some water while we wait?"

De-escalation Success: By focusing on David's underlying feelings of fear and loss of control rather than his threatening behavior, the nurse helped him calm down enough to cooperate with medical evaluation.

Trauma-Informed Communication

Many psychiatric patients have histories of trauma that affect how they perceive and respond to healthcare interactions (17). Trauma-informed communication recognizes this reality and adapts approaches to avoid re-traumatization.

Key Principles:

- Safety comes first—both physical and emotional
- Trustworthiness requires consistency and transparency
- Peer support provides hope and healing examples
- Collaboration includes patients in all decisions about their care
- Empowerment builds on patient strengths and resilience
- Cultural, historical, and gender considerations affect trauma responses

Practical Applications:

- Ask permission before touching patients for assessments
- Explain procedures and ask for consent throughout
- Offer choices whenever possible to restore sense of control
- Recognize that seemingly minor events might trigger trauma responses
- Avoid power struggles or authoritarian approaches
- Validate patient experiences without requiring detailed trauma disclosure

Case Study 3.3: Communicating with Non-English Speaking Patients

Carmen Rodriguez, a 45-year-old Spanish-speaking woman, presents with depression symptoms following her husband's death in a car accident three months ago. She speaks minimal English and appears withdrawn and tearful during the initial assessment.

Language Considerations: Professional interpreters are essential for accurate assessment and treatment planning. Family members, especially children, should not serve as interpreters for mental health issues due to confidentiality concerns and potential role conflicts.

Cultural Factors: In many Latino cultures, depression may be expressed through physical symptoms rather than emotional complaints. Carmen reports chronic headaches, fatigue, and stomach problems that began after her husband's death.

Therapeutic Approach with Interpreter:

Nurse (speaking to Carmen while maintaining eye contact): "Mrs. Rodriguez, I'm sorry for the loss of your husband. That must be incredibly difficult."

Interpreter (translates, then relays Carmen's response): "She says thank you. She says it's been very hard and she doesn't know how to go on without him."

Nurse: "Losing someone you love can make everything feel impossible. Can you tell me about the hardest parts of each day?"

Carmen (through interpreter): "Mornings are the worst. I wake up and forget he's gone for a moment, then I remember and the pain starts all over again. I can't eat or sleep."

Cultural Sensitivity: The nurse recognizes that Carmen's grief expression may differ from mainstream American patterns. Extended grieving periods are normal in many cultures, and family/community support systems play different roles.

Building Trust: By using professional interpretation services and showing respect for Carmen's cultural background, the nurse establishes a foundation for ongoing therapeutic work.

Technology-Mediated Communication

Telehealth has transformed psychiatric nursing practice, requiring adaptation of traditional communication skills to virtual platforms (18, 19). Video sessions present unique challenges and opportunities for therapeutic relationships.

Technical Considerations:

- Ensure reliable internet connection and backup plans

- Use HIPAA-compliant platforms for patient privacy

- Test audio and video quality before sessions

- Have phone contact information as backup

Therapeutic Adaptations:

- Position camera at eye level for natural interaction

- Use good lighting so patients can see your facial expressions

- Speak clearly and slightly slower than in person

- Pay attention to what's visible in your background

- Recognize limitations for certain assessments like gait or fine motor skills

Engagement Strategies:

- Begin sessions by checking in about the technology experience

- Be more intentional about verbal acknowledgments since subtle non-verbal cues are harder to see

- Ask patients to minimize distractions in their environment

- Use screen sharing for educational materials or assessment tools

- Plan shorter sessions to accommodate screen fatigue

Building Long-term Therapeutic Relationships

Psychiatric nursing often involves ongoing relationships that develop over weeks, months, or years. These extended relationships require special attention to boundaries, power dynamics, and professional development.

Boundary Management: Maintain professional limits while showing genuine care and concern. Share personal information only when it serves therapeutic purposes. Avoid dual relationships that could compromise your professional judgment or exploit patient vulnerability.

Power Awareness: Recognize the inherent power imbalance in nurse-patient relationships. Patients may be vulnerable due to mental illness, hospitalization, or life circumstances. Use this power responsibly to promote healing rather than personal gratification.

Professional Growth: Long-term therapeutic relationships can trigger countertransference—your emotional reactions to patients based on your own experiences. Regular supervision and self-reflection help you recognize and manage these responses constructively.

Communication Challenges and Solutions

Silent Patients: Don't rush to fill silence with questions or chatter. Comfortable silence can provide space for patients to gather thoughts or process emotions. When speaking, acknowledge the silence: "I notice you're taking time to think about this. That's okay."

Psychotic Patients: Don't argue with delusions or hallucinations, but don't pretend to see or hear them either. Focus on the feelings behind the symptoms: "It sounds like hearing those voices is really frightening for you."

Angry Patients: Stay calm and avoid taking anger personally. Often the anger masks fear, frustration, or helplessness. Acknowledge the emotion: "I can see you're really angry about this situation."

Manipulative Patients: Set clear, consistent boundaries and follow through on consequences. Don't get drawn into power struggles or feel guilty about maintaining limits. Remember that boundaries provide safety and structure that many patients need.

Documentation of Therapeutic Communication

Document significant conversations and patient responses, but avoid including excessive detail about your therapeutic techniques. Focus on patient statements, mood, behavior, and any safety concerns identified during interactions.

Effective Documentation Example: "Patient expressed hopelessness about his situation, stating 'Nothing ever gets better.' When asked about suicide, he denied current ideation but reported thinking about death frequently. Mood remained depressed throughout interaction despite supportive communication. Continues to engage appropriately in conversation and asks relevant questions about treatment options."

Avoiding Documentation Problems:

- Don't include your emotional reactions to patients

- Avoid judgmental language or personal opinions

- Don't document therapeutic techniques in detail unless relevant to outcomes

- Focus on objective observations and patient responses

Reflections on Human Connection

Therapeutic communication represents one of nursing's most sophisticated skills. It requires you to be fully present with another person's suffering while maintaining the emotional stability needed to provide effective care. This balance between engagement and professional distance takes time to develop.

Each patient teaches you something new about human resilience, courage, and the healing power of feeling understood. Even patients who initially seem resistant or difficult often respond to genuine empathy and respect. Your willingness to enter their world with compassion can become the turning point in their recovery journey.

The relationships you build through therapeutic communication will change you as much as they help your patients. You'll discover strengths you didn't know you had and learn lessons about life that textbooks can't teach. This is both the challenge and the privilege of psychiatric nursing practice.

Essential Takeaways for Practice:

- Therapeutic communication is a skill that improves with practice and self-reflection
- Cultural competence requires ongoing education and humility about your own biases
- De-escalation techniques can prevent violence and maintain therapeutic relationships
- Technology changes the medium but not the fundamentals of human connection
- Professional boundaries protect both patients and nurses
- Documentation should focus on patient responses and clinical outcomes
- Every interaction offers an opportunity to provide hope and healing

Chapter 4: Legal and Ethical Foundations

The intersection of law and ethics in psychiatric nursing creates some of the most challenging decisions you'll face in practice. A patient with schizophrenia refuses medication that could significantly improve their quality of life. An adolescent discloses suicidal plans but begs you not to tell their parents. A court orders treatment for someone who lacks insight into their mental illness. These scenarios require you to balance patient autonomy, beneficence, and legal requirements while maintaining therapeutic relationships.

Mental health law varies significantly by state and continues to evolve through legislation and court decisions. What remains constant is your responsibility to understand the legal framework governing your practice and to advocate for patients within that system. This chapter provides the foundation for making sound legal and ethical decisions in complex psychiatric situations.

Informed Consent and Capacity Assessment

Informed consent requires more than getting a signature on a form. Patients must understand the proposed treatment, its risks and benefits, available alternatives, and consequences of refusing treatment. In psychiatric settings, this process becomes complicated when mental illness affects decision-making capacity.

Capacity Assessment Components:

1. **Understanding**: Can the patient comprehend the information provided about their condition and treatment options?

2. **Appreciation**: Do they recognize how this information applies to their specific situation?

3. **Reasoning**: Can they weigh the risks and benefits of different options?

4. **Choice**: Are they able to communicate a consistent decision?

Capacity is decision-specific and can fluctuate with mental state changes. A patient might have capacity to consent to blood work but lack capacity for complex surgical decisions during the same hospitalization.

Case Study 4.1: Capacity Evaluation for Treatment Refusal

Michael Thompson, a 34-year-old man with bipolar disorder, is hospitalized during a severe manic episode. He's been awake for four days, spent his savings on expensive purchases, and drove recklessly before police brought him to the hospital. The psychiatrist recommends mood stabilizer medication, but Michael refuses, stating he feels "better than ever" and doesn't need treatment.

Capacity Assessment Process:

Understanding: When asked to explain his condition, Michael states, "They say I have bipolar disorder, but I'm just finally reaching my full potential. I don't need drugs to slow down my thinking."

Appreciation: He doesn't recognize that his elevated mood and decreased need for sleep represent symptoms of illness. He attributes his behavior to personal growth and enhanced abilities.

Reasoning: Michael can't weigh risks and benefits rationally because he doesn't acknowledge having a mental illness. He focuses only on feeling good and dismisses concerns about consequences.

Choice: He consistently refuses medication but his reasoning is based on impaired insight rather than rational decision-making.

Clinical Decision: Michael lacks capacity to refuse treatment during this acute manic episode. The treatment team can proceed with involuntary medication under emergency provisions while working to restore his decision-making abilities.

Ethical Considerations: This decision prioritizes beneficence (preventing harm) over autonomy (respecting choices) based on Michael's impaired capacity. As his symptoms improve with treatment, capacity should be reassessed and patient preferences honored when possible.

Involuntary Commitment Procedures

Civil commitment laws allow involuntary psychiatric hospitalization when specific criteria are met. These laws balance public safety concerns with individual rights, but their application varies significantly across jurisdictions.

Common Commitment Criteria:

- **Mental illness:** Must meet diagnostic criteria for a psychiatric condition

- **Dangerousness:** Risk of harm to self, others, or inability to care for basic needs

- **Lack of capacity**: Unable to make rational treatment decisions
- **Least restrictive alternative**: Outpatient treatment insufficient to ensure safety

Commitment Process:

1. **Emergency hold**: Brief detention (typically 72 hours) for evaluation
2. **Clinical assessment**: Comprehensive psychiatric and medical evaluation
3. **Legal hearing**: Court review of evidence and patient testimony
4. **Disposition**: Release, voluntary admission, or involuntary commitment

Case Study 4.2: Duty to Warn Scenario with Specific Threat

Sarah Martinez, a 28-year-old patient in outpatient therapy, reveals during a session that she plans to kill her ex-boyfriend who "ruined her life" by ending their relationship. She provides specific details about when and how she intends to carry out this plan and appears determined to follow through.

Legal Background: The Tarasoff decision established healthcare providers' duty to warn identifiable victims when patients make credible threats of violence. This duty overrides patient confidentiality when specific criteria are met.

Tarasoff Criteria:

1. **Specific threat**: Clear intent to harm an identifiable person
2. **Credible risk**: Patient has means and opportunity to carry out threat
3. **Imminent danger**: Threat likely to occur in near future

Required Actions:

1. **Warn the victim**: Contact ex-boyfriend directly about the threat
2. **Notify police**: Inform law enforcement of the danger
3. **Document thoroughly**: Record all actions taken and rationale
4. **Consider commitment**: Evaluate need for involuntary hospitalization

Therapeutic Considerations: The nurse maintains therapeutic relationship while fulfilling legal duties. Explain to Sarah why confidentiality must be breached and involve her in safety planning when possible.

Sarah's Response: "You said everything I told you was private! I trusted you!"

Therapeutic Response: "I understand you feel betrayed, and I'm sorry this is necessary. My first priority is keeping everyone safe, including you. Let's talk about other ways to deal with these angry feelings that won't put you at legal risk."

Confidentiality and Privacy Rights

HIPAA regulations provide the foundation for mental health confidentiality, but psychiatric nursing involves additional privacy considerations. Mental health information carries particular stigma, requiring extra protection beyond standard medical records.

Special Protections:

- **Psychotherapy notes**: Kept separate from medical records with additional consent requirements

- **Substance abuse treatment**: Federal regulations provide enhanced confidentiality

- **HIV/AIDS information**: Special disclosure restrictions in many states

- **Genetic information**: Emerging protections for genetic mental health risk factors

Permissible Disclosures Without Consent:

- **Medical emergencies**: When delay would endanger patient life

- **Mandatory reporting**: Child abuse, elder abuse, or other required reports

- **Court orders**: Judicial mandate for information disclosure

- **Public health**: Communicable disease reporting requirements

Case Study 4.3: Cultural Conflict in Treatment Decisions

Fatima Al-Hassan, a 22-year-old Muslim woman, is hospitalized for severe depression with psychotic features. Her family insists that her condition is spiritual rather than medical and refuses to consent to psychiatric medications. They want to take her home for religious healing ceremonies.

Cultural Considerations:

- Many cultures view mental illness through spiritual or supernatural frameworks

- Family involvement in medical decisions varies across cultures

- Religious practices may conflict with psychiatric treatment recommendations

- Immigration status might affect willingness to engage with authorities

Ethical Dilemmas:

- **Autonomy**: Whose decision matters—patient's, family's, or medical team's?

- **Beneficence**: What constitutes appropriate treatment in this cultural context?

- **Justice**: How do we provide culturally competent care while ensuring safety?

- **Non-maleficence**: Could forced treatment cause more harm than benefit?

Collaborative Approach: The treatment team arranges for a cultural liaison to help bridge differences between Western psychiatric care and the family's cultural beliefs. They explore ways to integrate religious practices with medical treatment.

Family Meeting Outcomes:

- Imam consultation supports medication as part of healing process

- Family agrees to trial of antipsychotic medication with close monitoring

- Religious practices incorporated into treatment plan where possible

- Discharge planning includes both psychiatric follow-up and spiritual support

Advance Directives in Mental Health

Psychiatric advance directives allow individuals to specify treatment preferences for future mental health crises when they might lack decision-making capacity. These documents help preserve patient autonomy during periods of illness-related incapacity.

Common Advance Directive Elements:

- **Medication preferences**: Specific drugs to use or avoid

- **Treatment settings**: Preferred facilities or providers

- **Crisis contacts**: Designated decision-makers or support persons

- **Intervention preferences**: Restraints, electroconvulsive therapy, hospitalization

Implementation Challenges:

- Legal recognition varies by state

- Healthcare providers may be unfamiliar with these documents

- Crisis situations may not allow time for document review

- Preferences made during wellness might not apply to current clinical situation

Ethical Decision-Making Framework

The four principles of biomedical ethics provide a structured approach to resolving ethical dilemmas in psychiatric nursing practice.

Autonomy: Respect for persons and their right to make decisions about their own lives. In psychiatry, this principle is complicated by conditions that may impair decision-making capacity.

Beneficence: Obligation to do good and promote patient wellbeing. This includes providing competent care and advocating for patient needs.

Non-maleficence: Duty to "do no harm" and avoid interventions that could cause more damage than benefit. In psychiatry, this includes considering side effects of medications and psychological effects of coercive interventions.

Justice: Fair distribution of benefits and burdens. This includes ensuring equal access to care regardless of diagnosis, social status, or ability to pay.

Applying Ethical Principles

When facing ethical dilemmas, work through each principle systematically:

1. **Identify the problem**: What specific ethical issue needs resolution?

2. **Gather facts**: What clinical, legal, and contextual information is relevant?

3. **Consider stakeholders**: Who is affected by potential decisions?

4. **Apply principles**: How do autonomy, beneficence, non-maleficence, and justice apply?

5. **Explore alternatives**: What different approaches are possible?

6. **Choose action**: Select the approach that best balances competing principles

7. **Evaluate outcomes**: Assess results and learn for future situations

Legal Documentation Requirements

Accurate documentation protects patients, supports clinical decision-making, and provides legal protection for nurses. Psychiatric documentation has special requirements due to the high-risk nature of mental health care.

Essential Elements:

- **Risk assessments**: Suicide, violence, and self-care capacity evaluations
- **Mental status findings**: Current psychological functioning
- **Medication administration**: Including refusals and patient responses
- **Behavioral observations**: Objective descriptions of patient actions
- **Interventions used**: Specific nursing actions and patient responses
- **Discharge planning**: Safety plans and follow-up arrangements

Documentation Best Practices:

- Write entries as soon as possible after events occur
- Use objective, descriptive language rather than interpretive statements
- Include direct quotes when relevant to clinical decisions
- Document all risk factors and protective factors identified
- Note any deviation from standard protocols and rationale
- Ensure entries are legible, dated, and signed with credentials

Mandatory Reporting Obligations

Psychiatric nurses have legal duties to report certain situations regardless of patient preferences or confidentiality concerns.

Child Abuse and Neglect:

- Physical, sexual, or emotional abuse
- Neglect of basic needs like food, shelter, medical care
- Exposure to domestic violence or substance abuse

Elder Abuse:

- Physical or emotional abuse

- Financial exploitation

- Neglect by caregivers

- Self-neglect when cognitive impairment present

Duty to Warn:

- Specific threats against identifiable victims

- Clear intent and means to carry out threats

- Imminent risk of violence

Public Health Threats:

- Communicable diseases

- Bioterrorism concerns

- Mass casualty incidents

Working with Legal Systems

Psychiatric nurses frequently interact with law enforcement, courts, and legal professionals. Understanding these relationships helps you advocate effectively for patients while meeting legal obligations.

Emergency Responses:

- Coordinate with police during crisis interventions

- Provide clinical information relevant to safety concerns

- Maintain therapeutic relationships when possible during legal proceedings

Court Involvement:

- Competency evaluations for criminal proceedings

- Civil commitment hearings

- Child custody evaluations

- Guardianship proceedings

Documentation for Legal Purposes:

- Records may be subpoenaed for court proceedings

- Testimony might be required in civil or criminal cases

- Maintain objectivity in all documentation

Professional Liability Considerations

Understanding your legal responsibilities helps prevent malpractice claims and protects your professional license.

Common Liability Areas:

- **Suicide prevention**: Failure to assess risk or implement safety measures

- **Medication errors**: Wrong drug, dose, or route administration

- **Patient falls**: Inadequate safety precautions for impaired patients

- **Confidentiality breaches**: Inappropriate disclosure of protected information

- **Informed consent**: Inadequate explanation of risks and alternatives

Risk Reduction Strategies:

- Follow institutional policies and procedures

- Document thoroughly and objectively

- Seek supervision when uncertain about decisions

- Maintain current knowledge through continuing education

- Report errors or near-misses through proper channels

Foundations for Ethical Practice

The legal and ethical challenges in psychiatric nursing require you to balance competing values while providing compassionate care. There are rarely perfect solutions—most situations involve choosing the approach that best serves patient wellbeing while respecting rights and meeting legal obligations.

Develop relationships with ethics committee members, legal counsel, and experienced colleagues who can provide guidance during difficult situations. Regular case consultation helps you learn from challenging experiences and improves your decision-making skills.

Remember that legal requirements provide the minimum standard for practice—ethical practice often demands more than what law requires. Your professional judgment and moral compass guide you toward actions that honor both the letter and spirit of ethical nursing care.

Core Practice Principles:

- Patient safety takes precedence over all other considerations

- Respect for persons includes those with impaired decision-making capacity

- Cultural competence requires understanding different worldviews about mental illness

- Documentation must be accurate, complete, and timely

- Professional consultation improves decision-making quality

- Legal requirements provide the framework for ethical practice

- Advocacy remains a fundamental nursing responsibility

Chapter 5: Care Planning Frameworks

Effective psychiatric care planning transforms assessment findings into actionable interventions that guide patients toward recovery goals. Unlike medical-surgical care plans that focus primarily on physiological problems, psychiatric care plans address the complex interplay between psychological, social, environmental, and spiritual factors that influence mental health.

The most successful care plans emerge from collaborative partnerships between patients, families, and treatment team members. These plans serve as roadmaps for recovery while remaining flexible enough to adapt as circumstances change. They provide structure for novice nurses while giving experienced practitioners a framework for organizing complex interventions.

NANDA-I/NIC/NOC System in Psychiatric Settings

The standardized nursing languages of NANDA International (NANDA-I), Nursing Interventions Classification (NIC), and Nursing Outcomes Classification (NOC) provide a systematic approach to psychiatric care planning (20, 21, 22, 23). These taxonomies help ensure consistent, evidence-based care while facilitating communication among healthcare providers.

NANDA-I Psychiatric Diagnoses commonly encountered include:

- Risk for Suicide related to hopelessness and social isolation

- Disturbed Thought Processes related to psychotic disorder

- Ineffective Coping related to inadequate social support

- Social Isolation related to fear of rejection

- Disturbed Sleep Pattern related to anxiety or medication side effects

NIC Interventions provide specific, research-based actions nurses can implement:

- Suicide Prevention: Environmental management, crisis intervention, safety planning

- Reality Orientation: Providing accurate information, promoting awareness of time and place

- Coping Enhancement: Teaching problem-solving skills, stress management techniques

- Socialization Enhancement: Facilitating interpersonal relationships and community connections

NOC Outcomes offer measurable indicators of patient progress:

- Suicide Self-Restraint: Demonstrates control over self-destructive impulses

- Cognitive Orientation: Maintains awareness of person, place, time, and situation

- Coping: Uses effective strategies to manage stressors

- Social Involvement: Participates in meaningful relationships and activities

Case Study 5.1: Comprehensive Care Planning for Major Depression

Jennifer Walsh, a 42-year-old marketing executive, is admitted to the psychiatric unit following a suicide attempt by overdose. She reports feeling "completely hopeless" since her divorce six months ago and states she "can't see any reason to keep living."

Assessment Findings:

- PHQ-9 score: 23 (severe depression)

- Sleep: 2-3 hours per night for past month

- Appetite: Reports 15-pound weight loss

- Social support: Minimal contact with friends or family since divorce

- Work functioning: On medical leave due to inability to concentrate

- Suicide risk: High intent, previous attempt, current ideation with method

Priority Nursing Diagnosis: Risk for Suicide related to hopelessness, social isolation, and previous attempt as evidenced by statements of worthlessness and recent overdose

Expected Outcomes (NOC):

- Suicide Self-Restraint: Patient will refrain from attempting self-harm during hospitalization (Score: Improve from 1 to 4 on 5-point scale)

- Hope: Patient will identify at least two reasons for living within 72 hours

- Depression Level: Patient will demonstrate decreased depressive symptoms as measured by PHQ-9 scores

Nursing Interventions (NIC):

Suicide Prevention:

- Conduct suicide risk assessment every shift using standardized tool

- Maintain constant visual supervision per protocol

- Remove potentially harmful objects from environment

- Engage patient in developing safety plan for discharge

Hope Instillation:

- Encourage expression of feelings about loss and life changes

- Help identify personal strengths and past coping successes

- Facilitate connection with supportive family members

- Explore future goals and aspirations

Mood Management:

- Monitor for medication side effects and therapeutic responses

- Encourage participation in unit activities and group therapy

- Teach relaxation techniques for anxiety management

- Assist with sleep hygiene practices

Implementation Example: Day 2: Jennifer participates in individual therapy session where she identifies her concern for her teenage daughter as a protective factor against suicide. She agrees to daily phone contact with daughter and expresses willingness to "try to get better for her sake." PHQ-9 score decreases to 19.

Day 5: Jennifer attends depression support group and shares her experience with other patients. She reports sleeping 5-6 hours last night and eating full meals for past two days. She begins working on discharge safety plan with social worker.

Day 7: Jennifer demonstrates ability to use coping skills independently and commits to outpatient therapy appointments. PHQ-9 score: 14. Discharged home with comprehensive safety plan and family support.

Evidence-Based Interventions

Modern psychiatric care planning incorporates interventions supported by rigorous research evidence. These interventions undergo continuous evaluation and refinement based on outcome studies and systematic reviews.

Cognitive-Behavioral Techniques help patients identify and modify dysfunctional thought patterns:

- Thought record keeping to track negative automatic thoughts
- Behavioral activation to increase pleasant activities
- Problem-solving skills training for life stressors
- Relaxation training for anxiety management

Psychoeducation Components provide patients and families with information about:

- Mental health condition symptoms and course
- Medication effects, side effects, and importance of adherence
- Warning signs of relapse and crisis management
- Community resources and support services

Motivational Interviewing Approaches enhance patient engagement:

- Exploring ambivalence about treatment
- Eliciting patient's own reasons for change
- Supporting self-efficacy and autonomy
- Rolling with resistance rather than confronting it directly

Case Study 5.2: Care Planning for Bipolar Disorder

Marcus Johnson, a 29-year-old teacher, is hospitalized during his third manic episode in two years. He stopped taking lithium three months ago because he "missed feeling creative and energetic." He presents with pressured speech, grandiose delusions about his teaching abilities, and hyperactivity that has kept him awake for four days.

Assessment Findings:

- Young Mania Rating Scale: 28 (severe mania)
- Insight: Poor recognition of illness or need for treatment

- Medication adherence: History of discontinuation during wellness periods
- Support system: Concerned parents and girlfriend
- Work status: Currently on administrative leave

Priority Nursing Diagnosis: Ineffective Health Management related to inadequate understanding of medication importance as evidenced by discontinuation of lithium and recurrent episodes

Expected Outcomes (NOC):

- Medication Adherence: Patient will demonstrate understanding of medication regimen and commit to adherence (Score: Improve from 2 to 4)
- Knowledge: Illness Care: Patient will verbalize understanding of bipolar disorder and treatment importance
- Mood Equilibrium: Patient will maintain stable mood within normal range

Nursing Interventions (NIC):

Medication Management:

- Assess understanding of bipolar disorder and medication purpose
- Provide education about lithium benefits and side effect management
- Discuss relationship between medication adherence and episode prevention
- Explore barriers to adherence and problem-solve solutions

Teaching: Disease Process:

- Use visual aids to explain mood cycling patterns
- Help patient identify personal triggers and early warning signs
- Involve family in education sessions
- Provide written materials for future reference

Mood Management:

- Monitor for medication response and side effects
- Encourage regular sleep schedule and stress management

- Facilitate discussion about balancing creativity with stability

- Support development of wellness plan for discharge

Implementation Progress: Week 1: Marcus begins to acknowledge that his elevated mood was problematic after reviewing consequences of his behavior (spending spree, inappropriate comments to students). He agrees to restart lithium.

Week 2: Marcus participates in psychoeducation group and creates personal early warning sign list. He identifies sleep disruption and increased goal-directed activity as his reliable early indicators.

Week 3: Marcus works with team to develop comprehensive wellness plan including mood monitoring, medication adherence strategies, and crisis contacts. He demonstrates understanding by teaching another patient about medication importance.

Recovery-Oriented Care Planning

Recovery-oriented approaches recognize that mental health recovery extends beyond symptom reduction to include hope, empowerment, and meaningful life engagement. Care plans incorporate patient-defined goals and emphasize strengths rather than deficits.

Recovery Principles:

- **Hope**: Recovery is built on belief that improvement is possible

- **Person-driven**: Patients direct their own recovery process

- **Many pathways**: No single approach works for everyone

- **Holistic**: Addresses all aspects of life, not just symptoms

- **Peer support**: People with lived experience provide unique assistance

- **Relational**: Recovery happens in community contexts

- **Cultural**: Approaches must be culturally relevant

- **Trauma-informed**: Recognizes widespread impact of trauma

- **Strengths-based**: Builds on existing capacities and resilience

Case Study 5.3: Recovery-Focused Planning for Schizophrenia

David Kim, a 34-year-old man with schizophrenia, has been homeless for six months since losing his job and apartment. He experiences persistent auditory hallucinations but has good insight into his condition and wants to "get my life back together."

Patient-Identified Goals:

1. "I want my own place to live"

2. "I want to work again, even part-time"

3. "I want the voices to bother me less"

4. "I want to reconnect with my sister"

Assessment of Strengths:

- Good insight into mental illness

- Motivated for treatment

- Previous work history in food service

- Basic computer skills

- Family member willing to provide support

Recovery-Focused Care Plan:

Goal 1: Stable Housing

- Connect with housing specialist for supported housing options

- Assist with housing applications and documentation

- Develop household management skills

- Plan for transition from shelter to independent living

Goal 2: Vocational Rehabilitation

- Referral to supported employment program

- Skills assessment for job placement

- Interview preparation and resume development

- Accommodation planning for workplace success

Goal 3: Symptom Management

- Medication optimization with psychiatrist
- Coping skills for auditory hallucinations
- Stress management techniques
- Regular monitoring and adjustment

Goal 4: Family Reconnection

- Family therapy sessions to address relationship concerns
- Communication skills training
- Gradual increase in contact frequency
- Support for sister's understanding of schizophrenia

Implementation Approach: David works with case manager to prioritize goals and develop timeline. Housing becomes first priority since stable living situation supports other goals. Peer support specialist with lived experience of homelessness provides mentorship and practical advice.

Six-month outcomes: David moves into supported housing, begins part-time work at restaurant, reports decreased distress from hallucinations, and has weekly contact with sister.

Interprofessional Collaboration

Modern psychiatric care involves multiple disciplines working together to address complex patient needs. Effective care planning requires coordination among team members with different expertise and perspectives.

Core Team Members:

- **Nurses**: 24-hour patient care, medication administration, crisis intervention
- **Psychiatrists**: Diagnosis, medication management, medical clearance
- **Social Workers**: Discharge planning, community resources, family therapy
- **Psychologists**: Psychological testing, individual and group therapy
- **Occupational Therapists**: Functional assessment, life skills training

- **Peer Support Specialists**: Shared experience, hope, practical guidance

Collaboration Strategies:

- **Regular team meetings**: Weekly rounds to review progress and adjust plans
- **Shared documentation**: Electronic records accessible to all team members
- **Clear role definition**: Understanding each discipline's scope and expertise
- **Conflict resolution**: Processes for addressing disagreements about care
- **Patient involvement**: Including patients in team meetings when possible

Quality Metrics and Outcome Measurement

Effective care planning includes specific, measurable outcomes that track patient progress and treatment effectiveness. These metrics support quality improvement efforts and evidence-based practice development.

Clinical Outcome Measures:

- Standardized assessment scores (PHQ-9, GAD-7, BPRS)
- Functional status improvements
- Medication adherence rates
- Crisis intervention frequency
- Rehospitalization rates

Patient-Reported Outcomes:

- Quality of life measures
- Treatment satisfaction scores
- Recovery goal achievement
- Hope and empowerment scales
- Perceived social support

System-Level Indicators:

- Length of stay trends

- Discharge disposition patterns

- Follow-up appointment attendance

- Emergency department utilization

- Community tenure stability

Technology Integration in Care Planning

Electronic health records and specialized software increasingly support psychiatric care planning through decision support tools, outcome tracking, and care coordination features.

Electronic Care Planning Benefits:

- Standardized assessment tools with automatic scoring

- Evidence-based intervention recommendations

- Outcome tracking and trending over time

- Automated reminders for reassessment and follow-up

- Communication platforms for team coordination

Challenges and Considerations:

- Learning curves for new technology adoption

- Privacy and security concerns with sensitive mental health data

- Integration challenges between different software systems

- Need for backup procedures when technology fails

- Ensuring technology enhances rather than replaces therapeutic relationships

Synthesis and Application

Effective psychiatric care planning requires integration of multiple frameworks, evidence-based interventions, and collaborative approaches. The most successful plans balance structure with flexibility, incorporating standardized tools while remaining responsive to individual patient needs and preferences.

As you develop care planning expertise, remember that plans serve as guides rather than rigid prescriptions. Patients' conditions change, new information emerges, and circumstances evolve. Regular reassessment and plan modification demonstrate responsive, patient-centered care.

The transition from novice to expert in care planning involves developing pattern recognition skills that help you anticipate patient needs and potential complications. This expertise comes through experience, mentorship, and continuous learning about evidence-based practices.

Fundamental Planning Principles:

- Patient goals drive all planning decisions

- Evidence-based interventions provide the foundation for quality care

- Recovery orientation emphasizes hope and empowerment

- Interprofessional collaboration maximizes expertise utilization

- Outcome measurement guides plan modifications

- Technology supports but never replaces clinical judgment

- Cultural competence ensures relevant and acceptable interventions

Care planning represents both science and art—applying research evidence while honoring individual patient experiences and preferences. Your ability to develop effective plans will determine much of your success as a psychiatric nurse and directly influence patient outcomes and recovery trajectories.

Final Reflections

These foundational chapters establish the groundwork for competent psychiatric nursing practice. The journey from understanding case-based learning principles to developing comprehensive care plans requires patience, practice, and commitment to lifelong learning.

Each patient encounter offers opportunities to refine your assessment skills, improve your therapeutic communication, navigate legal and ethical challenges, and create meaningful care plans that support recovery. The frameworks presented here provide structure for your developing expertise while encouraging the flexibility needed for individualized, culturally competent care.

Remember that psychiatric nursing affects both patients and practitioners profoundly. Your willingness to engage authentically with human suffering while maintaining professional boundaries creates the foundation for healing relationships. The legal and ethical principles guide your practice, while evidence-based interventions ensure you provide the most effective care possible.

As you progress through your career, these fundamentals will evolve and deepen through experience, continuing education, and professional development. The patients you serve will teach you lessons about resilience, hope, and human connection that textbooks cannot capture. This is both the challenge and the privilege of psychiatric nursing practice.

Key Takeaways from These Foundations

- Case-based learning accelerates the development of clinical reasoning skills essential for psychiatric nursing practice

- Systematic assessment using standardized tools and clinical observation provides the foundation for all nursing interventions

- Therapeutic communication skills can be learned and improved through practice, self-reflection, and mentorship

- Legal and ethical frameworks guide decision-making in complex situations while protecting both patients and practitioners

- Comprehensive care planning integrates evidence-based interventions with patient preferences and recovery goals

- Technology supports but cannot replace the human connection central to psychiatric nursing care

- Cultural competence requires ongoing self-examination and commitment to understanding diverse worldviews

- Professional development involves continuous learning about best practices, legal requirements, and ethical principles

Chapter 6: Inpatient Psychiatric Unit Cases

The psychiatric unit operates like no other medical floor in the hospital. You might walk into a patient's room to find them speaking with invisible companions, or discover another patient refusing all medications because they believe the nursing staff is part of a government conspiracy. These aren't unusual days—they're Tuesday morning rounds on the acute psychiatric unit.

Working in this environment requires you to think differently about patient care. Medical-surgical patients usually want to get better and go home. Psychiatric patients might not recognize they're ill, may fear treatment more than their symptoms, or believe hospitalization represents punishment rather than help. Your success depends on building trust with people who have every reason to be suspicious of healthcare providers.

Case Study 6.1: First-Episode Psychosis in Young Adult

Marcus Chen arrives at the emergency department on a cold Tuesday evening, brought by campus security after his roommate called for help. The 19-year-old computer science major at State University has been awake for three days straight, convinced that his professors are monitoring his thoughts through the campus WiFi network.

Day 1: Emergency Admission

Marcus sits rigidly in the corner of the ED triage room, constantly checking his phone for "surveillance signals." His clothes are wrinkled and smell unwashed. Dark circles under his eyes suggest prolonged sleep deprivation. His speech comes in rapid bursts punctuated by long pauses where he appears to be listening to something only he can hear.

"They're using advanced algorithms to track student thoughts," Marcus explains to the triage nurse. "I figured out their system—that's why they want me here. To stop me from exposing them."

Initial Assessment Findings:

- **Appearance**: Disheveled, poor hygiene, hypervigilant
- **Behavior**: Suspicious, avoids eye contact, frequently checks phone
- **Speech**: Pressured at times, whispered responses to apparent voices
- **Thought Process**: Circumstantial with loose associations

- **Thought Content**: Paranoid delusions about surveillance, no expressed suicidal ideation

- **Perceptual Disturbances**: Auditory hallucinations ("voices giving warnings")

- **Insight**: No recognition of mental illness

Family Dynamics: Marcus's parents, recent immigrants from Taiwan, arrive within two hours. His mother cries while speaking rapidly in Mandarin. His father, a software engineer, asks detailed questions about "brain scans" and "chemical imbalances." Both parents express shame about their son's condition and worry about family reputation in their community.

Cultural Considerations: Traditional Chinese culture often attributes mental illness to spiritual imbalance, family shame, or personal weakness. The parents need education about psychosis as a medical condition while respecting their cultural framework for understanding illness.

Day 3: Medication Initiation

After 48 hours of observation and safety monitoring, Marcus shows no improvement in psychotic symptoms. The treatment team recommends starting risperidone, an atypical antipsychotic medication. Marcus initially refuses, stating the medication is "part of the surveillance system."

Therapeutic Approach: The nurse uses motivational interviewing techniques to explore Marcus's concerns about medication while building rapport.

Nurse: "You seem worried about taking this medication. Help me understand your biggest concern."

Marcus: "It'll cloud my thinking. Then I won't be able to protect myself from them."

Nurse: "So you're concerned about staying alert and safe. That makes sense. Can you tell me more about how you've been protecting yourself lately?"

Marcus: "I haven't slept—sleep makes you vulnerable. I check my phone constantly for their signals."

Nurse: "That sounds exhausting. How is the lack of sleep affecting you?"

Marcus (pausing): "I... I am really tired. And the voices are getting louder."

This conversation reveals that Marcus recognizes some distressing aspects of his current state. The nurse builds on this awareness rather than arguing with his delusions.

Medication Education: The psychiatrist explains risperidone in terms Marcus can understand: "This medication helps reduce the intensity of voices and intrusive thoughts. It won't change your personality or make you a different person. Many people find it helps them think more clearly."

Marcus agrees to try the medication for three days to "test its effects."

Day 7: Family Meeting

Marcus shows modest improvement after four days of antipsychotic treatment. The voices are less frequent and distressing, though his paranoid beliefs persist. The family meeting includes Marcus, his parents, the psychiatrist, social worker, and primary nurse.

Goals of Family Meeting:

1. Educate family about first-episode psychosis

2. Address cultural concerns and stigma

3. Plan for ongoing support after discharge

4. Discuss early warning signs and relapse prevention

Family Education Points:

- **Psychosis explanation**: "Psychosis is like a brain storm—chemicals get out of balance and cause symptoms like hearing voices or suspicious thoughts"

- **Prognosis**: "With proper treatment, many people with first-episode psychosis recover well and return to their normal activities"

- **Treatment importance**: "Medication helps prevent future episodes and reduces symptom severity"

- **Support role**: "Family support significantly improves recovery outcomes"

Cultural Bridge-Building: The social worker involves a bilingual community health worker who helps explain the condition in culturally relevant terms. This person also connects the family with other Chinese-American families who have experienced similar situations.

Day 14: Discharge Planning

Marcus demonstrates significant improvement after two weeks of treatment. His paranoid thoughts are less intense, voices occur only occasionally, and he acknowledges that he was "not thinking clearly" when admitted. He agrees to continue medication and outpatient treatment.

Discharge Criteria Met:

- **Safety**: No longer poses risk to self or others

- **Stability**: Psychotic symptoms significantly reduced

- **Insight**: Some recognition of illness and need for treatment

- **Support**: Family committed to ongoing involvement

- **Follow-up**: Accepts outpatient appointments

NANDA-I Care Plan Development (24):

Priority Nursing Diagnosis: Disturbed Thought Processes related to biochemical imbalance as evidenced by paranoid delusions and auditory hallucinations

Expected Outcomes:

- Patient will demonstrate decreased intensity of psychotic symptoms within one week

- Patient will express understanding of illness and treatment within two weeks

- Patient will participate in discharge planning and agree to outpatient follow-up

Nursing Interventions:

- Monitor mental status every shift using standardized assessment tools

- Administer antipsychotic medication as prescribed and monitor for side effects

- Provide reality orientation without arguing with delusions

- Educate patient and family about psychosis and treatment importance

- Facilitate cultural consultation to address family concerns

Evaluation: Marcus met all expected outcomes by discharge and continued outpatient treatment successfully.

Case Study 6.2: Bipolar Disorder with Dual Diagnosis

Sarah Williams, a 35-year-old high school English teacher and single mother of two young children, presents to the psychiatric unit in a severe manic episode complicated by cocaine use. She was brought by police after neighbors reported her playing loud music at 3 AM and shouting about "writing the great American novel."

Presentation on Admission: Sarah appears disheveled despite wearing expensive clothes she claims to have purchased that morning using her "future royalty advances." She speaks rapidly about her "literary genius" and plans to "revolutionize education through poetry." Her pupils are dilated, and she admits to using cocaine "for creative inspiration" over the past week.

Complexity Factors:

- **Single parenting**: Children currently with Sarah's mother, who is elderly and struggling to manage

- **Employment**: School administration aware of absence, job security uncertain

- **Substance use**: Cocaine use during manic episode increases medical and psychiatric risks

- **Legal issues**: Potential charges for disturbing the peace and child endangerment

Day 1-3: Medical Stabilization and Substance Withdrawal

Sarah's initial treatment focuses on medical stabilization as cocaine withdrawal overlaps with manic symptoms. She experiences increased irritability, depression, and drug cravings as the stimulant effects wear off.

Medical Monitoring:

- Cardiac assessment due to cocaine's cardiovascular effects

- Hydration and nutrition support (hasn't eaten regularly in days)

- Sleep medication to address severe insomnia

- Seizure precautions during acute withdrawal

Psychiatric Assessment:

- Young Mania Rating Scale score: 32 (severe mania)

- Substance use history: Occasional alcohol use, first cocaine use during current episode

- Medication history: No previous psychiatric medications

- Insight: Denies mental illness, attributes behavior to "artistic breakthrough"

Day 4-7: Medication Initiation and Stabilization

As cocaine clears Sarah's system, the team initiates mood stabilizer treatment. The psychiatrist chooses lithium due to its proven efficacy in acute mania and suicide prevention.

Medication Challenges: Sarah initially refuses all psychiatric medications, stating she needs to maintain her "creative edge." The treatment team uses several approaches:

1. **Education about creativity and mood stability**: Explaining that mood stabilizers often improve rather than impair creative functioning

2. **Collaboration in medication choice**: Involving Sarah in discussions about different options

3. **Addressing concerns**: Exploring specific fears about side effects or personality changes

Social Services Coordination: The social worker becomes involved immediately due to child welfare concerns. Sarah's behavior before admission (leaving children with elderly grandmother while using cocaine) triggers mandatory reporting requirements.

Child Protective Services Meeting:

- **Assessment**: Children are safe with grandmother but long-term plan needed

- **Requirements**: Sarah must maintain psychiatric treatment and pass random drug tests

- **Timeline**: 30-day review with possible return of children if treatment compliance demonstrated

- **Support**: Family preservation services offered to assist with transition

Day 8-12: Group Therapy and Skills Development

As Sarah's mood stabilizes, she begins participating in unit programming. Her insights during this period prove particularly valuable for understanding dual diagnosis treatment.

Substance Abuse Group: Sarah shares how manic symptoms made her more impulsive about drug use: "When I feel like I can do anything, cocaine seems like a good idea. It wasn't until I crashed that I realized how dangerous it was."

Bipolar Education Group: She learns about the relationship between mood episodes and poor decision-making. This knowledge helps her understand recent behaviors without excessive shame.

Parenting Group: Sarah works with other parents in treatment to develop strategies for maintaining custody while managing mental illness.

Day 13-17: Discharge Planning and Reality Testing

As discharge approaches, Sarah faces the reality of consequences from her manic episode. This period often triggers depression as patients confront damage done during elevated mood states.

Challenges Identified:

- **Financial**: Spent $8,000 on credit cards during manic spending spree
- **Employment**: Must meet with school administration to discuss job status
- **Housing**: Behind on rent due to irresponsible spending
- **Children**: Must demonstrate stability before custody return

Discharge Plan:

- **Outpatient psychiatrist**: Weekly appointments for medication monitoring
- **Individual therapy**: Cognitive-behavioral therapy focused on mood management
- **Substance abuse treatment**: Intensive outpatient program with random testing
- **Peer support**: Bipolar support group that includes other single parents
- **Case management**: Help with benefits applications and housing assistance

Three-Month Follow-up: Sarah maintains mood stability on lithium, completes substance abuse treatment, and regains custody of her children. She returns to teaching with workplace accommodations for medical appointments.

Case Study 6.3: Severe Depression with Suicide Attempt

James Rodriguez, a 45-year-old Army veteran, is admitted to the psychiatric unit following a serious suicide attempt by overdose. His wife found him unconscious in their garage with empty pill bottles and a suicide note expressing hopelessness about his PTSD symptoms and inability to "be the man I used to be."

Military Cultural Context: James served three tours in Afghanistan as a combat medic. Military culture emphasizes strength, self-reliance, and emotional control—values that can conflict with seeking mental health treatment. Many veterans view mental health problems as personal weakness rather than service-related injuries.

Presentation and Assessment:

- **Physical status**: Medically cleared after 24-hour ICU stay for overdose

- **Mental status**: Severe depression with psychomotor retardation, minimal eye contact

- **Suicide risk**: High lethality method, detailed plan, strong intent

- **PTSD symptoms**: Nightmares, flashbacks, hypervigilance, emotional numbing

- **Social functioning**: Isolated from friends, strained marriage, unemployed

Day 1-5: Crisis Stabilization and Safety

James remains on constant observation due to high suicide risk. Initial interactions are minimal—he responds to questions with single words and spends most time lying in bed facing the wall.

Building Therapeutic Rapport: The primary nurse, also a veteran, uses this shared experience to establish connection without violating professional boundaries.

Nurse: "I noticed your Army tattoo. What unit were you with?"

James (barely audible): "68W. Combat medic."

Nurse: "That's tough work. You saw a lot over there."

James (making brief eye contact): "Too much."

This exchange represents the first meaningful interaction James has with staff. The nurse avoids excessive questions but validates his military experience.

Risk Assessment Documentation:

- **Suicide ideation**: Reports persistent thoughts of death, rates intensity 8/10

- **Plan**: Considered multiple methods, access to firearms at home

- **Intent**: States he "failed" in his attempt and might try again

- **Protective factors**: Concern for wife, some ambivalence about dying

- **Risk level**: High, requires constant supervision

Day 6-10: Medication Response and Therapy Engagement

James begins taking sertraline (an SSRI with good evidence for PTSD) and prazosin (for trauma-related nightmares). Initial medication response is minimal, which is expected with antidepressants.

Trauma-Informed Care Approach: Staff use trauma-informed principles recognizing that many interventions can trigger PTSD symptoms:

- Ask permission before entering personal space

- Explain procedures before implementing them

- Offer choices when possible to restore sense of control

- Avoid restraints or forced medications unless absolutely necessary

Group Therapy Participation: James initially refuses all groups but eventually attends a veterans-only PTSD group led by a veteran therapist. This specialized group addresses military-specific trauma experiences.

Family Involvement: James's wife Maria attends family therapy sessions. She reports feeling "like I'm walking on eggshells" and expresses her own need for support. The social worker connects her with a spouse support group.

Day 11-18: Technology Integration and Discharge Planning

James shows gradual improvement in mood and engagement. The treatment team develops a comprehensive discharge plan that includes telehealth components to address common barriers veterans face in accessing ongoing care (25, 26).

Telehealth Follow-up Planning: Many veterans live in rural areas with limited mental health resources or have difficulty traveling to appointments due to PTSD symptoms. Telehealth services help address these barriers:

- **Psychiatry appointments**: Monthly video sessions for medication management

- **Individual therapy**: Weekly telehealth sessions with trauma specialist

- **Group therapy**: Online veteran support groups that meet twice weekly

- **Crisis support**: 24/7 veteran crisis line with immediate access to counselors

Technology Training: Staff teach James to use the tablet provided by the VA for telehealth appointments. They practice connecting to sessions and troubleshoot potential technical problems.

Safety Planning: James works with his therapist to develop a detailed safety plan:

1. **Warning signs**: Sleep disruption, increased isolation, drinking alcohol

2. **Coping strategies**: Deep breathing, calling his sponsor, physical exercise

3. **Support people**: Wife, veteran buddy, therapist

4. **Professional contacts**: Psychiatrist, therapist, crisis line numbers

5. **Environmental safety**: Guns locked in safe with wife holding key

Discharge Outcomes: James leaves the hospital with significantly reduced suicide risk and commitment to ongoing treatment. His PHQ-9 score decreased from 23 to 16, and he reports hopefulness about recovery for the first time in months.

Six-Month Follow-up: James maintains regular telehealth appointments, participates actively in online veteran support groups, and reports no suicidal ideation. He begins volunteer work with a veteran service organization, finding meaning in helping other veterans access mental health care.

Understanding Inpatient Psychiatric Nursing

These three cases illustrate the complexity and diversity of inpatient psychiatric nursing. Each patient presents unique challenges requiring individualized approaches while maintaining safety as the primary concern.

Common Threads:

- **Crisis stabilization**: All three patients required immediate safety interventions

- **Medication management**: Each case involved careful medication selection and monitoring

- **Family involvement**: Support systems played critical roles in treatment success

- **Cultural competence**: Effective care required understanding diverse backgrounds

- **Discharge planning**: Successful transitions required comprehensive community connections

Nursing Skill Development: Working with these patient populations accelerates your development of:

- **Therapeutic communication** skills for building trust with suspicious or hopeless patients

- **Risk assessment** abilities to recognize subtle changes in safety status

- **Cultural competence** for working with diverse populations

- **Family education** techniques for involving support systems in treatment

- **Crisis intervention** skills for managing psychiatric emergencies

Professional Growth Opportunities: Inpatient psychiatric nursing offers unique chances to witness human resilience and recovery. Patients who arrive in crisis often leave with hope, skills, and connections that transform their lives. Your role in facilitating these transformations makes the challenges worthwhile.

The intensity of this work requires strong self-care practices and professional support. Regular supervision, peer consultation, and personal therapy when needed help maintain the emotional stability required for effective patient care.

Practical Applications for New Nurses

Building Therapeutic Relationships:

- Start with small, achievable interactions rather than trying to solve all problems immediately

- Listen more than you speak, especially during initial encounters

- Validate emotions while maintaining appropriate boundaries

- Use patient strengths and interests as building blocks for engagement

Managing Safety Concerns:

- Trust your instincts about patient safety—err on the side of caution

- Document all risk factors and protective factors thoroughly

- Communicate concerns clearly with team members

- Follow unit protocols consistently while adapting to individual needs

Working with Families:

- Include families in treatment planning from the beginning

- Provide education about mental illness and treatment options

- Address cultural concerns and misconceptions respectfully

- Connect families with community support resources

Professional Development:

- Seek mentorship from experienced psychiatric nurses

- Participate in continuing education about mental health conditions

- Join professional organizations like the American Psychiatric Nurses Association

- Maintain your own mental health through self-care practices

Bridge to Emergency Practice

The skills you develop in inpatient psychiatric nursing transfer directly to emergency department and crisis intervention work. Understanding how to quickly assess mental status, build rapport with distressed patients, and coordinate crisis interventions prepares you for the fast-paced environment of psychiatric emergencies.

The next chapter examines how these same principles apply when patients present in acute crisis situations requiring immediate intervention and rapid decision-making.

Essential Learnings for Professional Practice

- Inpatient psychiatric nursing requires balancing safety concerns with therapeutic relationship building

- Cultural competence significantly affects treatment engagement and outcomes

- Family involvement improves treatment adherence and recovery prospects

- Technology integration expands access to ongoing mental health care

- Comprehensive discharge planning prevents readmissions and supports community tenure

- Professional self-care is necessary for maintaining effectiveness in high-stress environments

- Therapeutic communication skills can be learned and improved through practice and feedback

- Risk assessment accuracy improves with experience and systematic documentation

Chapter 7: Emergency Department Psychiatric Emergencies

The emergency department at 2 AM presents a different world than the controlled environment of the psychiatric unit. Patients arrive in crisis—actively suicidal, psychotic, intoxicated, or violently agitated. You have minutes rather than days to assess safety, build rapport, and make critical decisions about treatment and disposition. The stakes are high, resources are limited, and families are often as frightened as the patients themselves.

Emergency psychiatric nursing requires you to think quickly while remaining calm, gather essential information efficiently, and provide therapeutic intervention in a chaotic environment. Your assessment skills determine whether patients receive appropriate care, and your communication abilities can de-escalate situations that might otherwise require restraints or sedation.

Case Study 7.1: Adolescent Mental Health Crisis

Taylor Johnson, a 16-year-old high school junior, arrives at the emergency department on a Friday evening accompanied by their frantic mother. Taylor's arms show fresh superficial cuts, and they're wearing clothes that don't match their birth-assigned gender. Their mother discovered the self-harm after finding bloody tissues in Taylor's bathroom.

Presentation Assessment: Taylor sits hunched forward, hoodie pulled up, avoiding eye contact with both mother and staff. They respond to questions with single words or silence. Their mother does most of the talking, alternating between worried inquiries about Taylor's safety and frustrated comments about their "recent behavior changes."

Initial Triage Findings:

- **Physical**: Multiple superficial lacerations on both forearms, cleaned and bandaged at home

- **Mental status**: Withdrawn, tearful, reports feeling "hopeless and trapped"

- **Suicide risk**: Active ideation but denies current intent or plan

- **Gender dysphoria**: Reports persistent discomfort with birth-assigned gender

- **Family conflict**: Increasing tension at home about gender identity

LGBTQ+ Considerations in Emergency Care: Working with LGBTQ+ youth requires special attention to language, confidentiality, and safety concerns. These patients face higher rates of depression, anxiety, and suicide attempts compared to their peers.

Inclusive Care Approaches:

1. **Language**: Use patient's preferred name and pronouns consistently

2. **Privacy**: Discuss confidentiality limits and mandatory reporting requirements

3. **Safety**: Assess for family rejection, school bullying, and social isolation

4. **Resources**: Connect with LGBTQ+-affirming mental health services

Building Rapport with Taylor: The emergency nurse begins by addressing Taylor directly rather than speaking only with their mother.

Nurse: "Hi Taylor. I'm Chris, and I'll be working with you tonight. I know this is probably not how you wanted to spend your Friday evening."

Taylor (slight smile): "Definitely not."

Nurse: "Can you help me understand what pronouns you'd like me to use?"

Taylor (looking up): "They and them, please."

Nurse: "Thanks for letting me know. That helps me talk with you more comfortably."

This brief exchange establishes respect for Taylor's identity and begins building trust.

Family Dynamics Assessment: The nurse speaks privately with Taylor's mother to understand family dynamics while Taylor receives medical evaluation for their cuts.

Mother: "I don't know what's happening to my daughter. Six months ago, she was normal, and now she wants to be called by a different name and use different pronouns. I'm trying to be supportive, but I'm scared she's going to hurt herself worse."

Nurse: "It sounds like you love Taylor very much and you're worried about their safety. That's completely understandable. These changes can feel overwhelming for families."

Mother: "I just want my child to be safe and happy. But I don't understand any of this."

Education and Support: The nurse provides brief education about gender dysphoria while validating the mother's concerns:

- Gender identity differences are not mental illness or parenting failures

- Family support significantly improves outcomes for LGBTQ+ youth

- Professional counseling can help both Taylor and family navigate this process

- Self-harm often results from distress rather than attention-seeking

Crisis Intervention and Safety Planning: The nurse meets with Taylor privately to assess suicide risk and develop a safety plan.

Safety Assessment:

- **Ideation**: "Sometimes I think about dying, especially when my parents argue about me"

- **Intent**: "I don't really want to die—I just want the pain to stop"

- **Method**: Has considered overdose but hasn't researched specifics

- **Access**: Parents keep medications locked, no firearms in home

- **Protective factors**: Supportive friend group, favorite teacher, pet dog

Safety Plan Development: Taylor works with the nurse to identify coping strategies and support resources:

1. **Warning signs**: Feeling "trapped," family arguments, social rejection

2. **Coping skills**: Texting supportive friends, listening to music, drawing

3. **Support people**: Best friend Alex, teacher Ms. Rodriguez, school counselor

4. **Professional contacts**: Crisis text line, local LGBTQ+ youth center

5. **Environment**: Remove sharp objects from bedroom, parents check in nightly

Disposition and Follow-up: Taylor doesn't meet criteria for involuntary hospitalization but needs intensive outpatient support. The emergency team coordinates referrals to:

- **Adolescent therapist** with LGBTQ+ specialization

- **Family therapy** to improve communication and support

- **Support group** for transgender youth

- **Primary care provider** experienced with gender-affirming care

Three-Month Outcome: Taylor engages successfully in therapy, self-harm episodes decrease significantly, and family relationships improve through education and counseling support.

Case Study 7.2: Geriatric Delirium vs. Dementia

Mary O'Brien, a 78-year-old nursing home resident, arrives at the emergency department via ambulance after becoming increasingly confused and agitated over the past two days. The nursing home staff report she tried to hit a aide during personal care and has been calling out for her deceased husband.

Presentation Challenges: Mary appears disoriented and frightened. She repeatedly asks for "Patrick" (her husband who died five years ago) and seems to recognize her surroundings as her childhood home. Her speech is clear but confused in content. She's pulling at her hospital gown and trying to get out of bed.

Differential Diagnosis Considerations: Distinguishing between delirium and dementia in elderly patients requires careful assessment, as both conditions can present with confusion and behavioral changes.

Delirium Characteristics:

- Acute onset (hours to days)
- Fluctuating consciousness and attention
- Often reversible with treatment of underlying cause
- Associated with medical illness, medications, or environmental changes

Dementia Characteristics:

- Gradual onset (months to years)
- Progressive cognitive decline
- Generally irreversible
- Memory loss is primary feature

Comprehensive Assessment: The emergency nurse gathers information from multiple sources to understand Mary's baseline functioning and recent changes.

Nursing Home Report:

- **Baseline**: Mild dementia, generally pleasant and cooperative
- **Recent changes**: Started three days ago with urinary symptoms
- **Current medications**: Includes newly prescribed antibiotic for UTI
- **Behavior changes**: Increased confusion, agitation during personal care

- **Physical symptoms**: Decreased appetite, possible low-grade fever

Medical Evaluation Findings:

- **Urinalysis**: Positive for urinary tract infection
- **Vital signs**: Low-grade fever (100.2°F), otherwise stable
- **Blood work**: Mild dehydration, elevated white blood cell count
- **Medication review**: Recent antibiotic addition, no other changes

Non-pharmacological Intervention Strategies: Rather than immediately using chemical or physical restraints, the nursing team implements behavior management techniques appropriate for confused elderly patients.

Environmental Modifications:

- **Lighting**: Adequate lighting to reduce shadows and misperceptions
- **Noise**: Minimize loud sounds and overhead pages
- **Orientation**: Clock and calendar visible, staff introduce themselves frequently
- **Familiar items**: Allow Mary to hold her purse or other comfort objects

Communication Approaches:

- **Simple language**: Short, clear sentences with concrete concepts
- **Validation**: Acknowledge emotions without arguing with confused content
- **Redirection**: Guide attention to pleasant topics or activities
- **Patience**: Allow extra time for processing and responses

Restraint Alternatives: Physical restraints often worsen confusion and agitation in elderly patients. The team uses alternative approaches:

Bed Alarm: Alerts staff when Mary attempts to get up independently **Frequent Monitoring**: Staff check on Mary every 15 minutes **Family Presence**: Daughter stays with Mary when possible **Comfort Items**: Stuffed animal and family photos reduce anxiety **Toileting Schedule**: Regular bathroom breaks prevent discomfort

Therapeutic Communication Example: Mary: "I need to go home. Patrick is waiting for me."

Nurse: "You're worried about Patrick. He must be very important to you."

Mary: "He's my husband. We've been married 52 years."

Nurse: "That's a long, wonderful marriage. Tell me about Patrick."

Mary (calming slightly): "He's so handsome. We met at a church dance..."

This approach validates Mary's emotions and memories without correcting her confusion about Patrick's death, which would likely cause distress.

Treatment and Resolution: Mary's delirium improves significantly after 48 hours of antibiotic treatment for her UTI. Her confusion decreases, and she returns to baseline functioning. The nursing home implements strategies to prevent future delirium episodes, including:

- Routine UTI screening

- Hydration monitoring

- Medication review protocols

- Staff education about delirium recognition

Case Study 7.3: Substance-Induced Psychosis

Ahmad Hassan, a 28-year-old construction worker, is brought to the emergency department by police after coworkers reported bizarre behavior at the job site. Ahmad was found dismantling electrical equipment while claiming it contained "listening devices" and became aggressive when supervisors tried to stop him.

Presentation and Assessment: Ahmad appears hypervigilant and agitated. His pupils are dilated, his heart rate is elevated, and he's sweating despite normal room temperature. He speaks rapidly about government surveillance and insists that his coworkers are "part of the conspiracy."

Substance Use History: Police found methamphetamine paraphernalia in Ahmad's truck. Coworkers report he's been acting "different" for the past week—staying late at work, talking excessively, and expressing paranoid ideas about management.

Cultural and Religious Considerations: Ahmad practices Islam and is currently observing Ramadan, which involves fasting from sunrise to sunset. This creates several considerations for his care:

Fasting Concerns:

- Medication timing must accommodate religious observance
- Dehydration from fasting may worsen methamphetamine effects
- Blood draws and IV fluids present religious considerations
- Food and water must be offered only during permitted hours

Cultural Factors:

- Family involvement expectations in Middle Eastern cultures
- Potential shame associated with drug use and mental health treatment
- Prayer needs and access to Islamic chaplain services
- Modesty concerns during medical examination and care

De-escalation Approach: Ahmad's agitation and paranoid thoughts require careful de-escalation to prevent violence and avoid need for restraints or forced medication.

Environmental Management:

- **Staff**: Limit number of people in room to avoid crowding
- **Positioning**: Nurse maintains safe distance with clear exit path
- **Stimulation**: Reduce bright lights and loud noises that worsen agitation
- **Space**: Provide adequate room for pacing and movement

Verbal De-escalation Techniques: **Nurse**: "Ahmad, I can see you're really concerned about your safety right now."

Ahmad: "You people don't understand! They're everywhere, watching everything I do!"

Nurse: "That sounds really frightening. Help me understand who you're worried about."

Ahmad: "The government, my boss, maybe even some of you. I can't trust anyone."

Nurse: "Feeling like you can't trust anyone must be really scary and exhausting."

Ahmad (slightly less agitated): "It is. I haven't slept in days because I have to stay alert."

Building Therapeutic Connection: The nurse acknowledges Ahmad's religious observance to show respect for his cultural identity:

Nurse: "I noticed you're observing Ramadan. That takes a lot of dedication and discipline."

Ahmad: "Yes, it's important to my faith. But this situation..." (trails off)

Nurse: "Your faith seems to give you strength. Would it help to speak with an imam or chaplain?"

Ahmad: "Maybe. I'm not sure what's happening to me."

This response suggests Ahmad has some insight into his altered mental state, which provides an opening for therapeutic intervention.

Medical Management: Methamphetamine intoxication requires both medical and psychiatric management:

Medical Monitoring:

- **Cardiovascular**: Continuous cardiac monitoring for arrhythmias
- **Hyperthermia**: Temperature monitoring and cooling measures if needed
- **Hydration**: IV fluids while respecting religious considerations
- **Seizure risk**: Monitoring and precautions during acute intoxication

Psychiatric Stabilization: Ahmad initially refuses all medications, believing they're part of the surveillance plot. The team uses several approaches:

Education: Explaining that medication will help reduce the frightening thoughts and sensations **Collaboration**: Involving Ahmad in medication decisions when possible **Religious considerations**: Ensuring medications don't conflict with religious practices **Family involvement**: With Ahmad's consent, contacting his brother for support

Chemical Restraint Considerations: If Ahmad became violent and posed immediate danger, chemical restraint might be necessary. However, the team successfully avoids this through:

- Consistent use of de-escalation techniques
- Respecting cultural and religious concerns
- Involving trusted family members in care
- Providing adequate space and minimal stimulation

Resolution and Follow-up: Ahmad's psychotic symptoms resolve as methamphetamine clears his system over 24-48 hours. He expresses remorse about his behavior and agrees to substance abuse treatment. The emergency team coordinates:

- **Substance abuse evaluation** and treatment referral

- **Primary care follow-up** for ongoing health management

- **Employee assistance program** referral through his construction company

- **Imam consultation** to address religious concerns about drug use

One-Month Follow-up: Ahmad successfully enters outpatient substance abuse treatment and maintains employment with regular drug testing. His psychotic symptoms don't recur, confirming substance-induced rather than primary psychotic disorder.

Emergency Psychiatric Nursing Principles

These three cases demonstrate core principles of emergency psychiatric nursing that apply across different patient populations and presentations.

Rapid Assessment Skills: Emergency psychiatric nurses must quickly gather essential information while building therapeutic rapport. This requires:

- **Prioritizing safety** assessment for patient, staff, and public

- **Identifying chief concerns** that brought patient to emergency care

- **Gathering collateral information** from family, friends, or other providers

- **Assessing mental status** systematically despite time constraints

- **Recognizing medical causes** of psychiatric symptoms

Cultural Competence in Crisis: Emergency situations don't allow time for extensive cultural education, but basic cultural competence improves outcomes:

- **Ask about preferences** for language, religious practices, and family involvement

- **Respect cultural values** while maintaining safety and treatment standards

- **Use interpreters** when language barriers exist

- **Involve cultural liaisons** or chaplains when available

- **Adapt interventions** to fit cultural frameworks when possible

De-escalation Expertise: Managing agitated or psychotic patients safely requires specialized communication skills:

- **Remain calm** and speak slowly in a low voice
- **Validate emotions** without agreeing with delusional content
- **Offer choices** when possible to restore sense of control
- **Avoid arguing** with psychotic thoughts or challenging beliefs directly
- **Use supportive presence** rather than excessive verbal intervention

Family and Caregiver Support: Families often experience their own crisis when loved ones have psychiatric emergencies:

- **Provide information** about what's happening and what to expect
- **Address immediate concerns** about safety and treatment
- **Educate about mental health** conditions and treatment options
- **Connect with resources** for ongoing support and education
- **Involve in treatment planning** when appropriate and with patient consent

Professional Development in Emergency Settings

Working emergency psychiatric cases accelerates your skill development in several key areas:

Clinical Judgment: The fast pace forces you to make decisions quickly while considering multiple factors **Communication**: You learn to establish rapport rapidly with diverse, distressed populations **Crisis Intervention**: Repeated exposure to psychiatric emergencies builds confidence and competence **Cultural Competence**: Emergency departments serve diverse populations requiring cultural adaptability **Interdisciplinary Collaboration**: You work closely with physicians, social workers, security, and community providers

Self-Care in High-Stress Environments: Emergency psychiatric nursing can be emotionally and physically demanding:

- **Debrief difficult cases** with colleagues or supervisors
- **Maintain physical fitness** to handle potential safety situations
- **Develop stress management** techniques for use during and after shifts

- **Seek professional support** when patient situations trigger personal issues

- **Balance caseload** with less acute patients when possible

Transition to Community Care

The emergency department represents just one point in the continuum of psychiatric care. Your assessment and intervention can determine whether patients successfully transition to outpatient treatment or require more intensive services.

Effective emergency care includes connecting patients with appropriate follow-up resources and ensuring they have the support needed to implement treatment recommendations. This bridge function makes emergency psychiatric nursing a critical component of the overall mental health system.

The next chapter explores how these principles apply in outpatient and community settings, where long-term therapeutic relationships support ongoing recovery and relapse prevention.

Core Competencies for Emergency Practice

- Rapid mental status assessment and risk evaluation skills are essential for safe emergency psychiatric care

- Cultural competence improves engagement and treatment outcomes across diverse populations

- De-escalation techniques can prevent the need for restraints and forced medications

- Family education and support are important components of emergency intervention

- Substance-induced psychiatric symptoms require both medical and psychiatric management

- Documentation must be thorough despite time pressures to ensure proper follow-up care

- Professional self-care is necessary to maintain effectiveness in high-stress emergency environments

- Coordination with community resources prevents repeated emergency department visits

Chapter 8: Outpatient and Community Mental Health

The weekly therapy appointment creates a different rhythm than the intensity of inpatient or emergency care. You watch patients make gradual progress over months rather than dramatic changes over days. This long-term perspective allows you to see recovery as a process—with setbacks, breakthroughs, and steady progress toward goals that patients define for themselves.

Community mental health nursing requires different skills than acute care settings. You become a coach rather than a crisis manager, helping patients develop tools for managing symptoms while building meaningful lives in their communities. Your office might be a traditional clinic, a patient's living room, or a community center meeting space.

Case Study 8.1: Treatment-Resistant Depression

Linda Thompson, a 52-year-old marketing executive, sits in the outpatient psychiatry clinic describing her frustration with yet another failed antidepressant trial. Over the past three years, she's tried six different medications with minimal improvement in her persistent depression symptoms.

Clinical History: Linda's depression began following her divorce three years ago but has persisted despite intensive treatment efforts. Her PHQ-9 scores consistently range from 16-20 (moderately severe to severe depression), and she reports significant impairment in work performance and social relationships.

Previous Treatment Attempts:

- **SSRIs**: Sertraline, escitalopram, fluoxetine (all caused sexual side effects with minimal mood improvement)

- **SNRIs**: Duloxetine, venlafaxine (moderate improvement but return of symptoms after 3-6 months)

- **Atypicals**: Bupropion caused anxiety; mirtazapine caused excessive weight gain

- **Therapy**: Individual CBT for 18 months with some skill development but persistent symptoms

Current Presentation: "I'm tired of trying medications that don't work or cause side effects I can't tolerate," Linda explains. "I function well enough to keep my job, but I feel like I'm just going through the motions of living. I want to try something different."

Innovation in Treatment Approach: Linda's psychiatrist discusses emerging treatment options, including psychedelic-assisted therapy, which shows promising results for treatment-resistant depression. Recent clinical trials demonstrate significant improvement rates for patients who haven't responded to traditional treatments.

Psychedelic-Assisted Therapy Evaluation: The treatment team evaluates Linda's eligibility for psilocybin-assisted therapy through a clinical trial:

Inclusion Criteria Met:

- Treatment-resistant depression (failed multiple medication trials)

- Stable medical health

- No history of psychotic disorders

- Ability to participate in intensive therapy process

- Strong support system for integration period

Exclusion Criteria Assessment:

- **Cardiovascular health**: EKG and stress test normal

- **Psychiatric history**: No bipolar disorder, psychosis, or active substance abuse

- **Medications**: Willing to taper antidepressants before treatment

- **Support system**: Sister and close friend available for post-session support

Preparation Phase (4 weeks): Linda attends weekly preparation sessions to:

- Learn about psilocybin effects and safety considerations

- Develop coping strategies for challenging experiences

- Set therapeutic intentions and goals

- Taper current antidepressant medication

- Strengthen support relationships

Treatment Sessions: Linda participates in two psilocybin-assisted therapy sessions in a controlled clinical setting:

Session 1: Linda experiences emotional processing of grief related to her divorce and childhood trauma. She reports feeling "connected to something larger than myself" and gains insights about self-worth and relationships.

Session 2: Three weeks later, Linda has a more introspective experience focused on self-compassion and acceptance. She describes feeling "lighter" and more hopeful about her future.

Integration Phase (12 weeks): Weekly therapy sessions help Linda integrate insights from her psychedelic experiences:

- **Week 1-2**: Processing emotional content and initial insights

- **Week 3-6**: Implementing behavioral changes based on new perspectives

- **Week 7-12**: Consolidating gains and developing long-term strategies

Telehealth Integration: Linda's treatment includes hybrid care combining in-person sessions for medication management and psychedelic therapy with telehealth sessions for ongoing support and integration work.

Telehealth Benefits:

- **Accessibility**: Reduces travel time for frequent appointments

- **Consistency**: Maintains therapeutic relationship between in-person sessions

- **Flexibility**: Accommodates Linda's demanding work schedule

- **Support**: Provides immediate access during challenging integration periods

Technology Considerations:

- **Platform security**: HIPAA-compliant video conferencing for privacy

- **Environment**: Linda creates private space at home for sessions

- **Backup plans**: Phone contact available if video connection fails

- **Assessment tools**: Online PHQ-9 and other measures between appointments

Three-Month Outcomes: Linda shows significant improvement following psychedelic-assisted therapy:

- **PHQ-9 score**: Decreased from 18 to 8 (mild depression range)

- **Functioning**: Improved work performance and renewed interest in social activities

- **Perspective**: Reports feeling "fundamentally different" about herself and her life

- **Relationships**: Begins dating and strengthens friendships

Six-Month Follow-up: Linda maintains improvement with monthly telehealth check-ins and occasional in-person sessions. She returns to previous activity levels and reports satisfaction with life quality.

Case Study 8.2: Schizophrenia in Community Setting

Robert Jackson, a 42-year-old man with chronic schizophrenia, has been homeless for eight months since losing his subsidized housing due to medication non-adherence and resulting symptom exacerbation. He receives services through the community mental health center's assertive community treatment (ACT) team.

Housing First Approach: Rather than requiring Robert to achieve sobriety or medication compliance before receiving housing assistance, the program provides stable housing as the foundation for other interventions (27, 28).

ACT Team Services: The multidisciplinary team provides intensive community-based services:

- **Psychiatrist**: Medication management and medical care

- **Nurse**: Health monitoring and medication administration

- **Social worker**: Benefits coordination and crisis intervention

- **Peer support specialist**: Shared experience and practical guidance

- **Substance abuse counselor**: Dual diagnosis treatment

- **Vocational specialist**: Employment support and job training

Initial Engagement Challenges: Robert initially distrusts the ACT team and refuses most services. His paranoid delusions include beliefs that mental health providers are government agents trying to control his thoughts through medication.

Engagement Strategies: The team uses patience and persistence to build trust:

- **Meet Robert where he is**: Services provided at homeless shelter or on the street

- **No demands**: Offer services without requiring immediate compliance

- **Basic needs focus**: Provide food, hygiene supplies, and medical care

- **Consistency**: Same team members visit regularly to build familiarity

- **Respect autonomy**: Honor Robert's choices while offering alternatives

Peer Support Integration: Marcus, a peer support specialist with lived experience of homelessness and schizophrenia, becomes key to engaging Robert.

Marcus's Approach: "I used to live under that same bridge," Marcus tells Robert during their third meeting. "I know how it feels when everyone thinks they know what's best for you."

Robert: "You really lived out here?"

Marcus: "For two years. I thought everyone was trying to hurt me, especially the mental health people. But I was tired of being cold and hungry all the time."

Robert: "What changed your mind?"

Marcus: "They didn't try to force me to take medication right away. They just helped me get a place to live and left me alone. After a while, I noticed I felt better when I took the medicine."

This conversation represents a breakthrough in Robert's willingness to consider services.

Housing Placement: After three months of engagement, Robert agrees to accept subsidized housing through the Housing First program:

Apartment Features:

- **Studio unit**: Private space with kitchen and bathroom

- **Support services**: On-site case management and peer support

- **Flexibility**: No sobriety or medication compliance requirements

- **Community**: Other residents with mental health conditions provide mutual support

Medication Management Evolution: Robert gradually becomes more willing to try psychiatric medications as his housing stabilizes:

Month 1-2: Refuses all medications but accepts vitamins and basic medical care **Month 3-4**: Agrees to try long-acting injectable antipsychotic "just once" to see effects **Month 5-6**:

Continues injections monthly, reports decreased paranoia and improved sleep **Month 7-12**: Adds mood stabilizer, achieves significant symptom reduction

Recovery Model Integration: The program emphasizes recovery principles that focus on hope, empowerment, and meaningful life engagement rather than just symptom management:

Hope: Robert begins to believe improvement is possible after seeing other residents' progress **Self-direction**: He chooses which services to accept and sets his own goals **Individualized**: Treatment plans adapt to Robert's preferences and cultural background **Strengths-based**: Focus on Robert's computer skills and desire to help others **Peer support**: Marcus and other residents provide encouragement and practical advice **Holistic**: Address housing, employment, relationships, and physical health **Trauma-informed**: Recognize impact of homelessness and mental illness stigma

Vocational Rehabilitation: As Robert's symptoms stabilize, he expresses interest in working again. The vocational specialist helps him:

- **Skills assessment**: Identify transferable abilities from previous data entry experience

- **Job coaching**: Practice interview skills and workplace social interaction

- **Supported employment**: Part-time position with on-site support and accommodation

- **Benefits counseling**: Understand how work income affects disability payments

Two-Year Outcomes: Robert maintains stable housing and shows significant functional improvement:

- **Housing**: Remains in same apartment with no eviction threats

- **Symptoms**: Minimal positive symptoms with good medication adherence

- **Employment**: Works 20 hours/week at nonprofit organization

- **Relationships**: Develops friendships with other residents and coworkers

- **Health**: Regular medical care and improved nutrition

His success illustrates how Housing First principles can break the cycle of homelessness and psychiatric hospitalization.

Case Study 8.3: Child and Adolescent ADHD

Maria Gonzalez, an 8-year-old third-grader, is referred to the community mental health center after her teacher reports persistent attention and behavioral problems that interfere with classroom learning. Her parents, both Spanish-speaking immigrants, express concerns about their daughter's academic performance and behavior at home.

Presentation and Assessment: Maria's teacher reports that she has difficulty sitting still, frequently interrupts others, and struggles to complete assignments. At home, her parents describe similar challenges with following directions and completing tasks like homework and chores.

Cultural Factors in Assessment: Hispanic family values and parenting styles can influence how ADHD symptoms are perceived and addressed:

Family Structure: Extended family involvement in childrearing decisions **Authority Respect**: Cultural emphasis on respecting adult authority and following rules **Academic Achievement**: High value placed on educational success and good behavior **Mental Health Stigma**: Reluctance to accept psychiatric diagnoses or medications **Language Barriers**: Need for Spanish-speaking providers and translated materials

Comprehensive Evaluation Process: The assessment includes multiple perspectives and cultural considerations:

Teacher Input:

- **Vanderbilt Assessment Scales**: Standardized rating forms completed by teacher

- **Classroom observation**: Direct observation of Maria's behavior during different activities

- **Academic performance**: Review of grades, test scores, and work samples

Parent Interview (conducted in Spanish):

- **Developmental history**: Pregnancy, birth, and early childhood milestones

- **Family history**: ADHD or other mental health conditions in relatives

- **Cultural perspectives**: Family beliefs about attention and behavior problems

- **Home environment**: Structure, routines, and behavioral management strategies

Medical Evaluation:

- **Physical exam**: Rule out hearing, vision, or other medical causes

- **Sleep assessment**: Sleep problems can mimic ADHD symptoms

- **Nutrition review**: Diet and eating patterns that might affect attention

Psychological Testing:

- **Cognitive assessment**: IQ testing to rule out learning disabilities

- **Attention measures**: Computerized testing of sustained attention and impulse control

- **Behavioral assessment**: Direct observation in clinical setting

Family Education and Engagement: Maria's parents need education about ADHD as a neurobiological condition rather than parenting failure or moral weakness:

Educational Components:

- **ADHD explanation**: Brain-based condition affecting attention and impulse control

- **Symptom description**: How inattention and hyperactivity appear in children

- **Treatment options**: Behavioral interventions, school accommodations, and medications

- **Prognosis**: Most children with ADHD can succeed with appropriate support

Cultural Bridge-Building: The clinic involves a bilingual family advocate who helps bridge cultural differences:

- **Cultural validation**: Acknowledging parents' concerns and values

- **Translation services**: Ensuring clear communication about diagnosis and treatment

- **Community resources**: Connecting family with Spanish-speaking support groups

- **Advocacy training**: Teaching parents to navigate school special education services

School Integration and IEP Development: Maria qualifies for special education services under the category "Other Health Impaired" due to her ADHD diagnosis:

IEP Team Members:

- **Parents**: Equal partners in educational planning

- **General education teacher**: Classroom instruction and behavior management

- **Special education teacher**: Specialized instruction and accommodations

- **School psychologist**: Assessment and behavioral intervention planning

- **School nurse**: Medication management during school hours

Educational Accommodations:

- **Seating arrangements**: Front of classroom to minimize distractions

- **Assignment modifications**: Breaking large tasks into smaller components

- **Time accommodations**: Extended time for tests and assignments

- **Behavioral supports**: Clear expectations and positive reinforcement systems

- **Communication tools**: Daily report cards between home and school

Medication Considerations: After trying behavioral interventions for three months with limited success, the family considers medication treatment:

Stimulant Medication Trial:

- **Methylphenidate**: Starting with low dose and gradual increases

- **Side effect monitoring**: Appetite, sleep, and growth tracking

- **School collaboration**: Teacher ratings to assess medication effectiveness

- **Cultural support**: Involving extended family in understanding medication benefits

Family Response to Medication: Maria's grandmother initially opposes medication use, believing behavioral problems should be addressed through stricter discipline. The treatment team provides education about ADHD as a medical condition and arranges for her to speak with other Hispanic families who have had positive medication experiences.

Six-Month Outcomes: Maria shows significant improvement with combined treatment approach:

- **Academic performance**: Grades improve from D's and F's to B's and C's

- **Classroom behavior**: Decreased disruptive behaviors and improved task completion

- **Home functioning**: Better compliance with rules and completion of chores

- **Self-esteem**: Increased confidence and willingness to participate in activities

- **Family relationships**: Reduced conflict and increased positive interactions

Long-term Planning: The treatment team develops a long-term plan for supporting Maria and her family:

- **Annual assessments**: Regular evaluation of medication effectiveness and side effects

- **School transitions**: Support for moving to middle school and high school

- **Skills development**: Social skills training and organizational coaching

- **Family support**: Ongoing education and connection with community resources

This case demonstrates how culturally responsive care can successfully engage families and improve outcomes for children with ADHD.

Community Mental Health Nursing Competencies

Working in outpatient and community settings requires specialized skills that differ from acute care nursing:

Long-term Relationship Building:

- **Trust development**: Building rapport over months rather than days

- **Boundary maintenance**: Managing longer relationships while staying professional

- **Motivation enhancement**: Helping patients maintain engagement during difficult periods

- **Recovery support**: Focusing on patient-defined goals rather than symptom elimination

Case Management Skills:

- **Resource coordination**: Connecting patients with housing, benefits, employment, and medical care

- **Advocacy**: Helping patients navigate complex systems and services

- **Crisis prevention**: Recognizing early warning signs and intervening before acute episodes

- **Team collaboration**: Working with multidisciplinary community providers

Cultural Competence:

- **Community understanding**: Learning about local cultural communities and resources

- **Language access**: Working with interpreters and translated materials

- **Family systems**: Understanding different cultural approaches to mental health and family involvement

- **Stigma reduction**: Addressing cultural barriers to mental health treatment

Technology Integration:

- **Telehealth proficiency**: Conducting effective therapy and medication management via video

- **Digital tools**: Using apps and online resources to support treatment goals

- **Documentation systems**: Managing electronic health records across multiple service sites

- **Communication platforms**: Coordinating care with team members and community providers

Professional Development in Community Settings

Community mental health offers unique opportunities for professional growth:

Autonomy: More independent practice and decision-making authority **Diversity**: Exposure to wide range of conditions, ages, and cultural backgrounds **Innovation**: Opportunities to implement new treatment approaches and programs **Advocacy**: Direct involvement in system change and policy development **Specialization**: Development of expertise in specific populations or treatment modalities

Challenges and Rewards:

- **Resource limitations**: Working within constrained budgets and service availability

- **Complex cases**: Managing patients with multiple diagnoses and social problems

- **Slow progress**: Measuring success over months and years rather than days

- **System navigation**: Helping patients access fragmented services

- **Professional isolation**: Less direct supervision and peer consultation than hospital settings

Connection to Specialized Settings

The skills developed in community mental health transfer to specialized populations and settings. Understanding long-term recovery processes, cultural competence, and resource coordination prepares you for working with older adults, medical patients, and individuals with substance use disorders.

The next chapter examines how these principles apply to specialized populations requiring adapted approaches and specialized knowledge.

Fundamental Practice Elements

- Outpatient care focuses on long-term recovery rather than crisis stabilization

- Innovation in treatment approaches offers hope for patients with treatment-resistant conditions

- Housing stability provides the foundation for mental health recovery in homeless populations

- Cultural competence is essential for engaging diverse communities in treatment

- School integration requires collaboration between mental health and educational systems

- Technology expands access to mental health services in community settings

- Recovery principles emphasize hope, self-direction, and meaningful life engagement

- Case management skills are essential for navigating complex community service systems

Chapter 9: Specialized Populations and Settings

Nursing practice in specialized psychiatric settings requires you to adapt core mental health skills to unique populations with distinct needs. An 82-year-old woman with Alzheimer's disease presents different challenges than a post-surgical patient experiencing steroid-induced psychosis or a healthcare professional struggling with opioid addiction. Each setting demands specific knowledge while maintaining the therapeutic principles that guide all psychiatric nursing.

These specialized environments often involve heightened ethical considerations, complex medical comorbidities, and regulatory requirements that don't exist in general psychiatric settings. Your ability to provide effective care depends on understanding these unique factors while maintaining the therapeutic relationships central to mental health nursing.

Case Study 9.1: Long-Term Care Dementia Management

William Chang, an 82-year-old retired professor with moderate Alzheimer's disease, has lived in the memory care unit for six months. Recently, his family and care staff report increasing agitation during evening hours (sundowning) and aggressive behavior during personal care activities.

Behavioral Symptom Presentation: William's symptoms follow a predictable pattern that has worsened over the past month:

- **Morning**: Generally calm and cooperative with basic care

- **Afternoon**: Becomes restless, paces hallways, asks repeatedly to "go home"

- **Evening**: Agitation peaks around 4-6 PM with increased confusion and anxiety

- **Personal care**: Resists bathing, changing clothes, often strikes out at staff

Regulatory Framework for Dementia Care: Centers for Medicare & Medicaid Services (CMS) guidelines strictly regulate psychotropic medication use in nursing homes (29, 30). The goal is to minimize chemical restraints while ensuring appropriate treatment for behavioral symptoms that pose safety risks.

CMS Requirements:

- **Documentation**: Detailed behavioral assessments before medication trials

- **Non-pharmacological interventions**: Must be attempted before medications

- **Monitoring**: Regular evaluation of medication effectiveness and side effects

- **Reduction attempts**: Periodic trials of medication decreases or discontinuation

- **Family involvement**: Informed consent and ongoing communication about treatment decisions

Comprehensive Behavioral Assessment: The nursing team conducts a detailed analysis of William's behavioral patterns to identify triggers and develop targeted interventions:

ABC Analysis (Antecedent-Behavior-Consequence):

- **Antecedents**: What happens before aggressive episodes?

- **Behaviors**: Specific actions and their intensity

- **Consequences**: How staff and environment respond to behaviors

Pattern Identification:

- **Timing**: Agitation increases during shift changes and meal preparation

- **Environment**: Loud noises and crowded spaces worsen symptoms

- **Physical**: Pain or discomfort from arthritis may trigger resistance to care

- **Social**: Unfamiliar staff members provoke more defensive responses

Non-Pharmacological Interventions: The team implements evidence-based strategies before considering medications:

Environmental Modifications:

- **Lighting**: Increased brightness during afternoon hours to reduce shadowing

- **Noise reduction**: Minimize overhead pages and equipment sounds during peak agitation times

- **Familiar objects**: William's family brings photographs and books from his academic career

- **Space design**: Clear pathways for pacing with comfortable seating areas

Person-Centered Care Approaches:

- **Life history**: Learn about William's preferences, routines, and meaningful activities

- **Communication**: Speak slowly, use simple sentences, maintain eye contact
- **Validation**: Acknowledge emotions without arguing with confused content
- **Redirection**: Guide attention to pleasant activities when agitation begins

Therapeutic Activities:

- **Music therapy**: Classical music from William's era reduces agitation
- **Reminiscence**: Looking through photo albums of his university teaching years
- **Physical activity**: Supervised walking during restless periods
- **Meaningful engagement**: Folding papers (mimicking academic work) provides purpose

Care Approach Modifications: Staff adapt personal care techniques to reduce resistance:

- **Timing**: Schedule bathing and care during William's calmest periods
- **Approach**: Same caregivers provide consistency and familiarity
- **Technique**: Break care tasks into smaller steps with frequent breaks
- **Communication**: Explain each step simply and wait for cooperation

Family Involvement and End-of-Life Planning: William's daughter struggles with watching her formerly brilliant father's cognitive decline. The team provides support and guidance about difficult decisions ahead:

Family Education:

- **Disease progression**: What to expect as Alzheimer's advances
- **Comfort care**: Shifting focus from curative to comfort-oriented interventions
- **Quality of life**: Defining meaningful activities and relationships
- **Medical decisions**: Advance directive discussions about feeding tubes, antibiotics, and hospitalization

Ethical Considerations:

- **Dignity**: Maintaining William's sense of self despite cognitive losses
- **Autonomy**: Honoring his preferences expressed before illness

- **Beneficence**: Balancing comfort with safety concerns

- **Non-maleficence**: Avoiding interventions that cause distress without clear benefit

Three-Month Outcome: Non-pharmacological interventions significantly reduce William's behavioral symptoms:

- **Sundowning**: Decreased from daily episodes to 2-3 times per week

- **Care resistance**: Improved cooperation with modified approaches

- **Family satisfaction**: Daughter reports feeling more comfortable with his care

- **Medication**: No psychotropic medications needed, avoiding potential side effects

This case demonstrates how person-centered, non-pharmacological approaches can effectively manage dementia-related behaviors while meeting regulatory requirements.

Case Study 9.2: Medical-Surgical Consultation

Patricia Davis, a 60-year-old retired nurse, is recovering from cardiac bypass surgery when she develops acute confusion and paranoid delusions on post-operative day three. The surgical team requests psychiatric consultation to evaluate her altered mental status and capacity to make treatment decisions.

Post-Operative Delirium Presentation: Patricia's family reports dramatic personality changes since surgery:

- **Cognitive**: Disoriented to time and place, difficulty following conversations

- **Behavioral**: Attempting to remove IV lines and monitoring equipment

- **Perceptual**: Claims nurses are trying to poison her through medications

- **Emotional**: Alternates between fearfulness and angry outbursts

Steroid-Induced Psychosis: Patricia received high-dose corticosteroids to reduce surgical inflammation. Steroid psychosis can develop within days of treatment initiation and presents with:

- **Mood symptoms**: Euphoria, depression, or mood lability

- **Psychotic symptoms**: Paranoid delusions, hallucinations, disorganized thinking

- **Cognitive changes**: Confusion, memory problems, poor judgment

- **Behavioral changes**: Agitation, aggression, or unusual behaviors

Differential Diagnosis Considerations: The psychiatric consultant must distinguish between multiple possible causes:

Post-Operative Delirium:

- **Anesthesia effects**: Residual medication impacts on brain function

- **Pain medications**: Opioids can cause confusion in older adults

- **Sleep disruption**: ICU environment prevents normal sleep cycles

- **Metabolic factors**: Electrolyte imbalances, dehydration, infection

Steroid Psychosis:

- **Dose-related**: Higher doses increase psychosis risk

- **Timing**: Usually develops within first week of treatment

- **Individual susceptibility**: Some patients more vulnerable than others

- **Reversibility**: Symptoms typically resolve with dose reduction

Medical Complications:

- **Infection**: Post-operative complications can cause delirium

- **Hypoxia**: Reduced oxygen levels affect brain function

- **Medication interactions**: Multiple drugs can interact to cause confusion

Interprofessional Collaboration: Managing Patricia's condition requires coordination among multiple specialties:

Cardiac Surgery Team:

- **Medical stability**: Ensuring surgical recovery remains on track

- **Medication review**: Identifying potentially problematic drugs

- **Family communication**: Updating relatives about complications

Psychiatry Consultation:

- **Differential diagnosis**: Distinguishing delirium from steroid psychosis

- **Treatment recommendations**: Medication and behavioral interventions

- **Capacity assessment**: Evaluating decision-making abilities

Nursing Coordination:

- **Safety management**: Preventing self-injury from confused behaviors

- **Environmental modification**: Reducing stimulation and reorientation

- **Family support**: Educating about temporary nature of symptoms

Capacity Assessment for Medical Decisions: Patricia needs to make decisions about ongoing cardiac care, but her mental state raises questions about decision-making capacity:

Capacity Evaluation:

- **Understanding**: Can Patricia comprehend information about her cardiac condition and treatment options?

- **Appreciation**: Does she recognize how this information applies to her situation?

- **Reasoning**: Can she weigh risks and benefits of different treatments?

- **Choice**: Is she able to communicate a consistent decision?

Assessment Findings:

- **Understanding**: Limited—Patricia has difficulty following explanations about her surgery

- **Appreciation**: Impaired—She believes staff are trying to harm rather than help her

- **Reasoning**: Significantly impaired—Cannot weigh treatment options rationally

- **Choice**: Inconsistent—Changes her mind frequently based on paranoid fears

Clinical Decision: Patricia lacks capacity for complex medical decisions during this acute episode. The team involves her healthcare proxy (her adult son) for major treatment decisions while continuing to include Patricia in discussions and respecting her preferences when possible.

Treatment Approach: The team implements a multi-modal intervention addressing both medical and psychiatric factors:

Steroid Management:

- **Dose reduction**: Gradual taper to minimum effective dose
- **Alternative medications**: Consider non-steroid anti-inflammatory options
- **Monitoring**: Close observation for symptom improvement

Delirium Prevention:

- **Sleep hygiene**: Reducing nighttime interruptions for non-essential care
- **Orientation**: Calendars, clocks, and familiar objects in room
- **Family presence**: Encouraging visits from familiar people
- **Mobility**: Early ambulation to prevent complications

Psychiatric Intervention:

- **Low-dose antipsychotic**: Quetiapine for severe paranoia and agitation
- **Monitoring**: Careful observation for cardiac effects given recent surgery
- **Non-pharmacological**: Reassurance, reality orientation, therapeutic presence

Resolution and Recovery: Patricia's symptoms improve gradually over five days as steroids are tapered and delirium resolves:

- **Day 1-2**: Continued confusion and paranoia despite interventions
- **Day 3-4**: Slight improvement in orientation, decreased agitation
- **Day 5**: Clear improvement, recognizes family members, rational conversation
- **Day 7**: Full resolution of psychotic symptoms, capacity restored

Lessons for Practice: This case illustrates important principles for psychiatric consultation in medical settings:

- **Multiple causation**: Medical patients often have several factors contributing to psychiatric symptoms
- **Collaboration**: Effective treatment requires coordination among multiple specialties
- **Temporary impairment**: Capacity can fluctuate and improve as medical conditions resolve
- **Family involvement**: Support systems play crucial roles during periods of incapacity

Case Study 9.3: Substance Use Treatment Center

Michael Park, a 30-year-old emergency department nurse, enters residential substance use treatment following intervention by his hospital's employee assistance program. He has been diverting opioid medications for his own use while struggling with depression and work-related stress.

Professional Considerations in Healthcare Worker Addiction: Healthcare professionals with substance use disorders face unique challenges that affect treatment planning and recovery:

Professional Identity Crisis: "I became a nurse to help people," Michael explains during his intake assessment. "Now I'm the patient everyone thinks is hopeless. How do I reconcile being a caregiver with being an addict?"

Shame and Stigma: Healthcare workers often experience intensified shame about addiction due to:

- **Professional expectations**: "Nurses should know better"
- **Patient care concerns**: Guilt about potentially compromising patient safety
- **Career consequences**: Licensing board investigations and employment restrictions
- **Peer judgment**: Concerns about colleagues' reactions and trust

Dual Diagnosis Assessment: Michael presents with both opioid use disorder and major depression, requiring integrated treatment for both conditions:

Substance Use History:

- **Onset**: Began using leftover patient medications after back injury two years ago
- **Progression**: Advanced to diverting medications during shifts
- **Consequences**: Near-miss medication errors, relationship problems, financial difficulties
- **Insight**: Recognizes he has a problem but struggles with feeling hopeless about recovery

Depression Evaluation:

- **PHQ-9 score**: 19 (moderately severe depression)

- **Symptoms**: Persistent sadness, sleep problems, concentration difficulties, worthlessness

- **Suicidal ideation**: Passive death wishes but no active plan

- **Functional impairment**: Difficulty performing job duties, social isolation

Medication-Assisted Treatment (MAT) Integration: The treatment team recommends buprenorphine for opioid use disorder management:

Buprenorphine Benefits:

- **Reduces cravings**: Helps manage physiological dependence

- **Improves functioning**: Allows patients to work and maintain relationships

- **Safety profile**: Lower overdose risk compared to full opioid agonists

- **Professional compatibility**: Enables return to healthcare practice with monitoring

Induction Process:

- **Withdrawal assessment**: Clinical Opioid Withdrawal Scale (COWS) monitoring

- **Timing**: Starting buprenorphine during mild to moderate withdrawal

- **Dosing**: Gradual titration to effective maintenance dose

- **Monitoring**: Daily assessment for first week, then less frequent

Integrated Treatment Approach: Michael's treatment addresses both substance use and depression simultaneously:

Individual Therapy:

- **Cognitive-behavioral therapy**: Addressing negative thought patterns and developing coping skills

- **Trauma processing**: Exploring work-related traumatic experiences that contributed to substance use

- **Professional identity work**: Rebuilding sense of professional self and exploring how recovery can enhance rather than diminish his nursing abilities

Group Therapy Components:

- **Healthcare professionals group**: Meeting with other nurses, doctors, and pharmacists in recovery

- **Dual diagnosis group**: Addressing the interaction between substance use and mental health

- **Process group**: General addiction recovery work with diverse professional backgrounds

Family Therapy: Michael's wife attends weekly sessions to address:

- **Trust rebuilding**: Working through betrayal and deception related to his addiction

- **Communication skills**: Learning to discuss recovery needs and challenges openly

- **Codependency patterns**: Addressing her tendency to enable his avoidance behaviors

- **Relapse prevention**: Developing family strategies for supporting long-term recovery

Professional Rehabilitation Planning: The treatment team works with the state nursing board and hospital administration to develop a return-to-work plan:

Nursing Board Requirements:

- **Practice monitoring**: Supervised nursing practice with restricted access to controlled substances

- **Random drug testing**: Frequent urine screens for two years

- **Support group attendance**: Mandatory participation in healthcare professionals recovery group

- **Therapy compliance**: Ongoing individual and group therapy requirements

Hospital Accommodation:

- **Modified duties**: Initially working in areas without controlled substance access

- **Peer support**: Partnering with colleague mentor who understands recovery process

- **Schedule flexibility**: Accommodating therapy appointments and recovery meetings

- **Gradual progression**: Increasing responsibilities as recovery stability demonstrated

Recovery Milestones and Outcomes:

30 Days: Michael completes residential treatment with improved mood (PHQ-9: 12) and stable on buprenorphine. He demonstrates understanding of recovery principles and commitment to ongoing treatment.

90 Days: Returns to work on modified duties with nursing board oversight. Continues outpatient therapy and maintains medication adherence. Relationship with wife shows improvement through ongoing counseling.

Six Months: Expands nursing responsibilities with continued monitoring. Depression symptoms minimal (PHQ-9: 6). Active in healthcare professionals recovery support group as peer mentor.

One Year: Full nursing practice restored with continued monitoring. Maintains recovery stability and strong family relationships. Considers specializing in addiction medicine to help other healthcare professionals.

Two Years: Completes nursing board monitoring requirements. Enrolls in addiction nursing certification program. Becomes advocate for addressing healthcare worker addiction through system-level interventions.

Lessons for Professional Practice: Michael's case highlights important considerations for healthcare worker addiction:

Early Intervention: Employee assistance programs can identify problems before patient safety is compromised **Integrated Treatment**: Addressing co-occurring mental health conditions improves substance use outcomes **Professional Support**: Recovery groups specifically for healthcare workers provide unique understanding and support **Regulatory Collaboration**: Working with licensing boards can facilitate safe return to practice **Stigma Reduction**: Successful recovery stories help reduce shame and encourage others to seek treatment

Specialized Setting Competencies

Working in specialized psychiatric settings requires adaptation of core nursing skills to unique populations and regulatory environments:

Regulatory Knowledge:

- **CMS guidelines**: Understanding federal requirements for psychotropic medication use in nursing homes

- **Joint Commission standards**: Meeting accreditation requirements for specialized units

- **Professional licensing**: Working with regulatory boards for healthcare professionals with substance use disorders

- **Legal requirements**: Mandatory reporting and consent procedures for specialized populations

Population-Specific Skills:

- **Geriatric assessment**: Distinguishing normal aging from pathological changes

- **Medical complexity**: Managing psychiatric symptoms in medically compromised patients

- **Professional dynamics**: Understanding unique challenges faced by healthcare workers with mental health conditions

- **Family systems**: Adapting interventions for different developmental stages and cultural contexts

Ethical Sensitivity:

- **Capacity assessment**: Evaluating decision-making abilities in cognitively impaired patients

- **Dual relationships**: Managing professional boundaries when treating colleagues

- **End-of-life care**: Balancing comfort with psychiatric symptom management

- **Confidentiality**: Protecting privacy in specialized treatment settings

Interdisciplinary Collaboration:

- **Medical teams**: Coordinating psychiatric care with ongoing medical treatment

- **Regulatory agencies**: Working with licensing boards and oversight organizations

- **Family systems**: Involving appropriate support persons in treatment planning

- **Community resources**: Connecting patients with specialized support services

Professional Development in Specialized Settings

Specialized psychiatric settings offer unique opportunities for advanced practice development:

Expertise Development: Deep knowledge of specific populations and conditions
Leadership Opportunities: Program development and quality improvement initiatives
Research Participation: Contributing to evidence base for specialized interventions
Advocacy Work: Influencing policy and practice standards for vulnerable populations
Teaching Roles: Educating other professionals about specialized care approaches

Challenges and Rewards:

- **Complex cases**: Managing multiple comorbidities and psychosocial factors

- **Regulatory oversight**: Navigating complex compliance requirements

- **Resource limitations**: Working within specialized program constraints

- **Ethical dilemmas**: Balancing autonomy with safety in vulnerable populations

- **Professional growth**: Developing expertise in niche areas of psychiatric nursing

Integration with Contemporary Issues

The specialized populations examined in this chapter connect directly to emerging issues in psychiatric nursing. Understanding how to work with older adults, medical patients, and healthcare professionals prepares you for contemporary challenges like climate anxiety, technology integration, and healthcare worker burnout.

The next chapters explore these contemporary issues and their impact on psychiatric nursing practice, building on the foundation of specialized care principles covered here.

Specialized Care Foundations

- Regulatory compliance is essential for safe and legal practice in specialized psychiatric settings

- Non-pharmacological interventions often provide effective alternatives to medication in vulnerable populations

- Interprofessional collaboration is crucial for managing complex medical and psychiatric comorbidities

- Professional identity issues require special attention when treating healthcare workers with mental health conditions

- Family involvement and education improve outcomes across all specialized populations

- Ethical considerations become more complex when treating patients with impaired decision-making capacity

- Cultural competence must be adapted to specific population needs and characteristics

- Technology integration can improve access to specialized mental health services

Synthesis and Moving Forward

These specialized settings demonstrate the breadth and complexity of contemporary psychiatric nursing practice. Each environment requires you to adapt fundamental skills while developing new competencies specific to unique populations and regulatory requirements.

The cases presented illustrate how core principles of therapeutic communication, assessment, and care planning apply across diverse settings while highlighting the specialized knowledge needed for effective practice. Your ability to work successfully in these environments depends on understanding both universal psychiatric nursing principles and population-specific considerations.

As healthcare continues to evolve, these specialized skills become increasingly important. The aging population will require more dementia care expertise. Medical advances create new opportunities for psychiatric consultation in complex medical cases. The opioid epidemic demands skilled professionals who can address healthcare worker addiction with compassion and clinical expertise.

Your professional development in psychiatric nursing benefits from exposure to these specialized settings, even if you ultimately choose to practice in general psychiatric environments. The skills and perspectives gained from working with diverse populations enhance your ability to provide culturally competent, ethically sound, and clinically effective care to all patients.

The next section of this textbook examines contemporary issues and emerging challenges in psychiatric nursing, building on these foundational skills to address current and future practice demands.

Chapter 10: Technology-Enhanced Psychiatric Care

The smartphone in your pocket carries more computing power than the room-sized computers that once filled entire buildings, yet many psychiatric patients still struggle to access basic mental health services. Technology promises to bridge gaps in care—reaching rural communities, providing 24/7 support, and offering innovative treatments that seemed like science fiction just decades ago. But technology alone can't heal the human heart or mend a broken spirit.

Your role as a psychiatric nurse now includes learning to use video platforms for therapy sessions, understanding virtual reality applications for exposure therapy, and helping patients navigate smartphone apps that track their moods and medications. This technological shift doesn't replace the therapeutic relationship—it expands your reach and adds new tools to your clinical practice.

Case Study 10.1: Telehealth for Rural Mental Health

José Martinez, a 24-year-old farmworker in rural Nebraska, drives forty-five minutes each way to reach the nearest mental health clinic. Between his demanding agricultural schedule and limited transportation options, he's missed more appointments than he's attended despite struggling with depression and anxiety that interfere with his work and relationships.

Rural Mental Health Barriers: José's situation reflects challenges faced by millions of Americans living in areas with severe mental health provider shortages:

Geographic Isolation:

- Nearest psychiatrist is 90 miles away with a six-month waiting list

- Mental health clinic only open three days per week

- Weather conditions often make travel dangerous or impossible

- No public transportation available

Economic Constraints:

- Hourly wages mean lost income for each appointment

- Vehicle maintenance costs for long-distance travel

- Limited health insurance coverage for mental health services

- Seasonal work patterns create income uncertainty

Cultural Factors:

- Traditional Latino culture emphasizes family problem-solving over professional help

- Language barriers with predominantly English-speaking providers

- Stigma about mental health treatment in rural communities

- Preference for face-to-face relationships over technological solutions

Technology Infrastructure Challenges: The clinic develops a hybrid care model after assessing José's technological capabilities and limitations:

Internet Assessment:

- José owns a smartphone with basic data plan

- Home internet connection is satellite-based with occasional outages

- Download speeds adequate for video calls but sometimes unstable

- No computer or tablet access

Technology Skills Evaluation:

- Comfortable with basic smartphone functions and text messaging

- Limited experience with video calling applications

- Willing to learn new technology if it improves access to care

- Prefers Spanish-language interfaces when available

Hybrid Care Model Development: The treatment team creates a flexible approach combining in-person and virtual services:

Initial Engagement (Month 1):

- First appointment conducted in-person to establish therapeutic relationship

- Technology training session using clinic equipment to practice video sessions

- Assessment of home environment for private video calling space

- Introduction to mood tracking app with Spanish language option

Maintenance Phase (Months 2-6):

- Video sessions every two weeks with bilingual therapist
- Monthly in-person appointments with psychiatrist for medication management
- Weekly check-ins via text message with care coordinator
- Access to crisis line with Spanish-speaking counselors

Crisis Contingency:

- Same-day video appointments available during crisis situations
- Protocol for emergency department coordination if needed
- Family member trained to assist with technology during crisis episodes
- Backup phone contact if video connection fails

Therapeutic Adaptations for Video Sessions: The therapist modifies traditional techniques for effective video delivery:

Environmental Considerations:

- José uses his bedroom for privacy during sessions
- Headphones provided to ensure confidentiality from family members
- Session timing adjusted to avoid peak internet usage hours
- Backup location identified in case of interruptions

Communication Modifications:

- Slower speech pace to accommodate potential audio delays
- More frequent verbal check-ins since subtle non-verbal cues are harder to observe
- Use of chat feature for sharing resources and homework assignments
- Screen sharing for educational materials and worksheets

Therapeutic Relationship Building: "I wasn't sure talking to someone on my phone would help," José admits during his fourth video session. "But having you check in with me every week makes me feel less alone out here."

Cultural Integration: The therapist incorporates José's cultural values into treatment:

- **Family involvement**: Including his wife in some sessions with his consent

- **Religious considerations**: Incorporating his Catholic faith into coping strategies

- **Work identity**: Acknowledging pride in agricultural work and seasonal rhythms

- **Language preference**: Conducting sessions in Spanish to improve comfort and expression

Digital Tools Integration: José learns to use smartphone applications that support his mental health goals:

Mood Tracking App:

- Daily ratings of mood, anxiety, and sleep quality

- Photo journal feature for documenting positive moments

- Medication reminder system with customizable alerts

- Data sharing with therapist for session preparation

Meditation App:

- Guided relaxation exercises in Spanish

- Short sessions designed for work breaks

- Offline download capability for areas with poor reception

- Progress tracking to maintain motivation

Resource Database:

- Local community resources and support groups

- Crisis contact information easily accessible

- Educational materials about depression and anxiety

- Links to Spanish-language mental health websites

Outcome Measurement: The team tracks José's progress using multiple digital and clinical measures:

Clinical Assessments:

- PHQ-9 scores completed monthly via secure online portal

- GAD-7 anxiety assessments during video sessions

- Functional impairment measures related to work and relationships

- Medication adherence tracking through app data

Technology Engagement:

- Video session attendance rates (90% compared to 40% for in-person only)

- App usage frequency and feature utilization

- Crisis line contact frequency and outcomes

- Patient satisfaction with technology-enhanced care

Six-Month Outcomes: José demonstrates significant improvement across multiple measures:

- **Depression symptoms**: PHQ-9 score decreased from 17 to 8

- **Anxiety management**: Reports improved coping with work stressors

- **Medication adherence**: Consistent use of antidepressant with app reminders

- **Functional improvement**: Better work performance and family relationships

- **Technology comfort**: Independently troubleshoots minor technical issues

José's Reflection: "I thought I'd have to choose between getting help and keeping my job. Now I can do both. The technology took some getting used to, but it's made getting help possible for someone like me."

This case demonstrates how thoughtful integration of technology can overcome traditional barriers to mental health care while maintaining therapeutic effectiveness.

Case Study 10.2: VR Therapy for PTSD

Ashley Brown, a 32-year-old combat veteran, has struggled with PTSD symptoms for three years since returning from deployment in Afghanistan. Traditional exposure therapy has been only partially successful, as she finds it difficult to engage with imagined scenarios or written exercises about her traumatic experiences.

Traditional Exposure Therapy Limitations: Ashley's previous treatment attempts illustrate common challenges with conventional PTSD interventions:

Imaginal Exposure Difficulties:

- "I can't get the images right in my head," Ashley explains
- Difficulty maintaining focus on traumatic memories during therapy sessions
- Avoidance behaviors that prevent full engagement with exposure exercises
- Limited ability to control or modify imagined scenarios

In-Vivo Exposure Barriers:

- Real-world exposure to triggers too intense and uncontrolled
- Safety concerns with exposing veterans to combat-related situations
- Geographic limitations for accessing relevant environments
- High cost and logistical challenges of real-world exposure

VR Exposure Therapy Protocol: The treatment team introduces virtual reality exposure therapy (VRET) as an innovative approach combining benefits of controlled exposure with realistic environments:

Technology Setup:

- **VR Headset**: High-resolution display with spatial audio for immersive experience
- **Biometric Monitoring**: Heart rate and skin conductance sensors to track physiological responses
- **Control Interface**: Therapist can adjust scenario intensity in real-time
- **Safety Features**: Immediate disconnection capability if distress becomes excessive

Evidence Base Review: Recent research demonstrates VRET effectiveness for PTSD treatment:

- **Randomized controlled trials** show equivalent or superior outcomes to traditional exposure therapy
- **Physiological studies** confirm that VR environments activate similar stress responses as real-world triggers
- **Neuroimaging research** reveals similar brain activation patterns during VR and real-world exposure

- **Meta-analyses** support VRET as evidence-based treatment for trauma-related disorders

Graduated Exposure Scenarios: Ashley's treatment progresses through increasingly challenging virtual environments:

Level 1: Safe Base Environment:

- Virtual recreation of secure military base with familiar sights and sounds
- Practice relaxation techniques while wearing VR equipment
- Build comfort with technology and therapist's voice guidance
- Establish baseline physiological responses

Level 2: Non-Combat Military Scenarios:

- Virtual convoy rides through peaceful countryside
- Interaction with virtual military personnel in safe contexts
- Practice coping skills in mildly stressful but non-threatening situations
- Gradual introduction to military vehicles and equipment

Level 3: Moderate Threat Environments:

- Virtual patrols in urban environments with ambient threat
- Sounds of distant explosions or gunfire without immediate danger
- Practice grounding techniques while maintaining VR engagement
- Therapist guidance for processing emotional responses

Level 4: High-Intensity Combat Scenarios:

- Virtual recreation of specific traumatic events with therapist control
- Ability to pause, modify, or exit scenarios as needed
- Processing of trauma memories with visual and auditory cues
- Integration of trauma narrative with corrective information

Nursing Role in VR Therapy: Ashley's primary nurse plays several important roles in successful VRET implementation:

Pre-Session Preparation:

- **Equipment check**: Ensuring VR hardware functions properly
- **Baseline assessment**: Measuring anxiety, heart rate, and blood pressure
- **Safety planning**: Reviewing grounding techniques and emergency procedures
- **Consent process**: Confirming Ashley's willingness to participate

During Session Support:

- **Physiological monitoring**: Tracking biometric data for safety and effectiveness
- **Communication facilitation**: Serving as liaison between Ashley and therapist
- **Crisis intervention**: Prepared to provide immediate support if needed
- **Environmental management**: Maintaining quiet, private space for sessions

Post-Session Care:

- **Debriefing support**: Helping Ashley process emotional responses to VR exposure
- **Coping skills application**: Reinforcing relaxation techniques learned during session
- **Safety assessment**: Evaluating need for extended observation or support
- **Documentation**: Recording session details and patient responses

Technology Integration Challenges: The team addresses several technical and clinical challenges during implementation:

Motion Sickness:

- Some patients experience nausea or dizziness with VR use
- Gradual acclimatization with shorter initial sessions
- Anti-nausea medications available if needed
- Alternative approaches for patients who can't tolerate VR

Technical Malfunctions:

- Backup equipment available in case of hardware failure
- Technician support for troubleshooting during sessions

- Manual alternatives prepared if technology becomes unavailable
- Regular equipment maintenance and updates

Therapeutic Relationship Maintenance:

- Ensuring technology enhances rather than replaces human connection
- Regular non-VR therapy sessions for relationship building
- Therapist presence and guidance throughout VR experiences
- Processing technology experiences within therapeutic context

Ashley's Progress Through Treatment:

Week 1-2: Technology acclimatization and safe environment exposure

- Initial anxiety about VR equipment decreases with practice
- Successfully completes 20-minute sessions in safe base environment
- Reports feeling "more in control" compared to imaginal exposure

Week 3-6: Progressive exposure to military environments

- Tolerates convoy scenarios with minimal distress
- Heart rate stabilizes more quickly after exposure sessions
- Begins identifying specific triggers and coping responses

Week 7-10: Trauma-specific scenario processing

- Engages with modified versions of traumatic experiences
- Able to "pause" scenarios when overwhelmed and resume when ready
- Processes trauma narrative with corrective information about survival and meaning

Week 11-12: Integration and generalization

- Applies coping skills learned in VR to real-world situations
- Reports decreased avoidance of trauma-related triggers
- Plans for post-treatment maintenance and continued progress

Treatment Outcomes: Ashley shows significant improvement across multiple PTSD symptom clusters:

- **Re-experiencing symptoms**: Decreased flashbacks and intrusive thoughts
- **Avoidance behaviors**: Increased willingness to engage in social situations
- **Negative cognitions**: Improved self-concept and outlook on future
- **Hyperarousal**: Better sleep quality and reduced startle responses

Technology Acceptance: "At first, I thought VR was just a gimmick," Ashley reflects. "But being able to control the experience—to face my memories when I'm ready and stop when I need to—that made all the difference. I could never do that with my actual memories."

Implementation Considerations for Other Sites: This case provides insights for implementing VR therapy in various psychiatric settings:

Equipment Requirements:

- Initial investment in VR hardware and software systems
- Ongoing technical support and maintenance needs
- Staff training for operation and troubleshooting
- Space requirements for safe VR therapy sessions

Staff Development:

- Training for therapists in VR-specific exposure protocols
- Nursing education about biometric monitoring and crisis intervention
- Technician support for equipment management
- Ongoing education about emerging VR applications

Patient Selection:

- Assessment for VR therapy appropriateness and contraindications
- Evaluation of technology comfort and acceptance
- Consideration of specific trauma types and treatment goals
- Alternative options for patients who can't tolerate VR

Technology Integration Principles

These cases illustrate core principles for successful technology integration in psychiatric care:

Patient-Centered Approach: Technology should serve patient needs rather than driving treatment decisions. José's hybrid model respected his cultural preferences while addressing access barriers. Ashley's VR therapy provided control and gradual exposure that traditional methods couldn't offer.

Therapeutic Relationship Preservation: Technology supplements but never replaces human connection in psychiatric care. Both cases maintained strong therapeutic relationships while using technology to overcome specific barriers or enhance treatment effectiveness.

Cultural and Individual Adaptation: Successful technology integration requires adaptation to individual patient characteristics, cultural values, and technological capabilities. One-size-fits-all approaches fail to maximize technology benefits.

Safety and Ethics Considerations: Technology use in psychiatric care requires attention to privacy, security, informed consent, and crisis management. Clear protocols ensure patient safety while maximizing treatment benefits.

Nursing Competencies for Technology-Enhanced Care

Modern psychiatric nurses need new skills to effectively integrate technology into practice:

Technical Proficiency:

- Basic troubleshooting for video conferencing and therapeutic apps
- Understanding of privacy and security requirements for digital health
- Ability to teach patients technology use and provide ongoing support
- Familiarity with emerging technologies like VR and artificial intelligence

Assessment Adaptation:

- Modified techniques for evaluating mental status via video
- Integration of digital data from apps and wearable devices
- Understanding limitations of remote assessment methods
- Crisis intervention protocols for technology-mediated care

Patient Education:

- Teaching technology skills to diverse patient populations

- Explaining benefits and limitations of digital mental health tools

- Supporting patients through technology-related frustrations

- Promoting digital literacy and safe technology use

Professional Development:

- Staying current with rapidly evolving mental health technologies

- Understanding evidence base for new technological interventions

- Maintaining professional boundaries in digital environments

- Advocating for equitable access to technology-enhanced care

Looking Ahead to Emerging Challenges

The technology skills you develop today prepare you for addressing emerging mental health challenges that require innovative solutions. Climate anxiety, social media-related disorders, and pandemic-related mental health issues all benefit from technology-enhanced interventions.

The next chapter examines these contemporary mental health challenges and how the technological tools discussed here can be adapted to address new forms of psychological distress.

Technology Integration Foundations

- Technology can overcome traditional barriers to mental health care access and engagement

- Virtual reality offers new possibilities for controlled exposure therapy and skills training

- Hybrid care models combining in-person and digital services maximize flexibility and effectiveness

- Cultural adaptation is essential for successful technology implementation across diverse populations

- Nurses play critical roles in technology integration, patient education, and safety monitoring

- Therapeutic relationships remain central even when enhanced by technological tools

- Professional development must include ongoing technology education and competency development

- Equity considerations ensure technology benefits reach underserved populations rather than widening gaps

Chapter 11: Emerging Mental Health Challenges

Your grandmother worried about war, economic depression, and polio. Your parents faced nuclear threats, social upheaval, and the HIV epidemic. Now you confront climate change, social media addiction, and global pandemics that reshape human psychology in ways previous generations never imagined. Each era brings unique mental health challenges that require nurses to adapt traditional skills while developing new interventions.

The patients you treat today present with conditions that didn't exist in textbooks from even a decade ago. Climate anxiety affects young people who see their planet heating up while politicians debate science. Healthcare workers develop moral injury from making impossible decisions during resource shortages. Adolescents attempt suicide after cyberbullying campaigns that follow them home through their smartphones.

Case Study 11.1: Climate Anxiety in Young Adults

Emma Wilson, a 21-year-old environmental studies student at a prestigious university, sits in your office describing a familiar pattern of anxiety and despair that seems to intensify with each climate report or extreme weather event. She tracks global temperature data obsessively and has stopped making long-term plans because she believes "civilization will collapse within my lifetime."

Presentation and Assessment: Emma's symptoms reflect a growing phenomenon affecting young people worldwide as they confront the reality of climate change (31, 32):

Anxiety Symptoms:

- Persistent worry about environmental catastrophe
- Physical symptoms including sleep disruption and appetite changes
- Panic attacks triggered by weather news or extreme temperature days
- Avoidance of climate-related media that paradoxically increases her anxiety

Depressive Features:

- Hopelessness about the future and personal life plans
- Guilt about her own carbon footprint despite minimal individual impact
- Anger at older generations for "destroying the planet"
- Social withdrawal from friends who "don't understand the urgency"

Functional Impairment:

- Academic performance declining despite high motivation
- Relationship conflicts over environmental issues
- Difficulty enjoying activities due to constant environmental worry
- Career indecision based on apocalyptic thinking

Activism Burnout: Emma has been involved in environmental activism since high school, but her commitment has become compulsive rather than empowering:

Compulsive Activism Patterns:

- Attending every climate protest and meeting, even when exhausted
- Checking environmental news multiple times daily despite increased distress
- Arguing with family and friends about environmental issues
- Feeling guilty about any non-environmental activities or enjoyment

Burnout Symptoms:

- Physical exhaustion from constant activity and worry
- Cynicism about the effectiveness of environmental action
- Reduced sense of personal accomplishment despite significant efforts
- Irritability and impatience with others' environmental awareness

Meaning-Focused Therapy Approach: The treatment team uses meaning-focused therapy principles to help Emma maintain environmental commitment while developing psychological resilience:

Core Principles:

- **Acceptance:** Acknowledging legitimate environmental concerns without minimizing them
- **Values clarification:** Identifying what matters most to Emma beyond environmental activism
- **Meaning-making:** Finding purpose and significance in environmental work

- **Resilience building**: Developing capacity to sustain long-term commitment without burnout

Therapeutic Interventions:

Session 1-3: Validation and Assessment Emma needs to feel heard and understood rather than told her concerns are "irrational":

Therapist: "Your worry about climate change isn't crazy—the science supports serious concern. Help me understand how this worry affects your daily life."

Emma: "Finally, someone who gets it! Most people think I'm overreacting, but the data is terrifying. I can't stop thinking about what the world will look like in 30 years."

Therapist: "It sounds like carrying this knowledge feels overwhelming. How do you balance staying informed with taking care of yourself?"

Emma: "I don't think I do balance it. I feel guilty if I'm not constantly working on climate issues."

Session 4-8: Meaning Exploration The therapist helps Emma explore what environmental work means to her beyond anxiety reduction:

Values Identification Exercise:

- **Core values**: Justice, future generations, natural beauty, scientific truth
- **Meaningful activities**: Research, education, community organizing, policy advocacy
- **Personal strengths**: Intelligence, persistence, communication skills, leadership ability
- **Life domains**: Career, relationships, health, spirituality, community

Meaning-Making Questions:

- "What drew you to environmental work originally?"
- "How has your advocacy made a difference, even in small ways?"
- "What would you want to contribute to environmental solutions over your lifetime?"
- "How can you honor your environmental values while also caring for yourself?"

Session 9-12: Resilience and Sustainability Emma learns to maintain environmental commitment while developing psychological sustainability:

Sustainable Activism Strategies:

- **Boundaries**: Limiting news consumption to specific times and sources
- **Self-care**: Regular exercise, sleep, and non-environmental activities
- **Community**: Connecting with other environmentally minded people for support
- **Efficacy focus**: Choosing specific, achievable environmental actions

Cognitive Reframing Techniques:

- **Temporal perspective**: Balancing urgency with long-term sustainability
- **Sphere of influence**: Focusing energy on areas where she can make a difference
- **Collective action**: Recognizing individual limitations while appreciating group power
- **Hope cultivation**: Identifying positive environmental trends and solutions

Community Resource Integration: Emma connects with local environmental groups that emphasize both action and member wellbeing:

Environmental Action Groups:

- **Local chapter of Citizens Climate Lobby**: Policy-focused advocacy with structured approach
- **University sustainability office**: Campus-based projects with measurable outcomes
- **Community garden collective**: Hands-on environmental work with social benefits
- **Climate grief support group**: Processing emotions with others who share similar concerns

Therapeutic Activities:

- **Nature immersion**: Regular time outdoors to reconnect with what she's working to protect
- **Environmental journalism**: Writing about solutions and positive developments
- **Mentoring**: Teaching younger students about environmental issues and activism

- **Policy research**: Contributing academic work to environmental solution development

Treatment Outcomes: After three months of meaning-focused therapy, Emma shows significant improvement:

Anxiety Reduction:

- GAD-7 score decreased from 18 to 10 (severe to moderate anxiety)
- Sleep quality improved with consistent bedtime routine
- Panic attacks reduced from weekly to rare occurrences
- Able to engage with environmental news without overwhelming distress

Functional Improvement:

- Academic performance returns to previous high levels
- Relationships improve as environmental discussions become less confrontational
- Career planning resumes with realistic timeline and goals
- Increased enjoyment of non-environmental activities without guilt

Sustainable Activism:

- Continues environmental work but with better boundaries and self-care
- Leadership role in campus sustainability office provides concrete impact
- Connects with other environmentally committed peers for mutual support
- Plans graduate studies in environmental policy with career goals intact

Emma's Reflection: "I realized that burning myself out wasn't helping the planet—it was just making me miserable and ineffective. I can still care deeply about climate change while also taking care of myself and enjoying my life. Actually, I think I'm a better activist now because I'm not constantly overwhelmed."

Case Study 11.2: Social Media and Adolescent Mental Health

Aiden Kim, a 15-year-old high school sophomore, presents with worsening depression and anxiety that his parents attribute to "too much screen time." Aiden spends 6-8 hours daily on various social media platforms and has recently experienced cyberbullying related to his physical appearance and academic performance.

Digital Environment Assessment: Aiden's online experience illustrates common patterns affecting adolescent mental health:

Platform Usage:

- **Instagram**: Primary platform for social comparison and image-focused content

- **TikTok**: Short-form video consumption, often late into the night

- **Snapchat**: Communication with peers and social status tracking

- **Discord**: Gaming communities with both positive and negative interactions

- **Twitter**: News consumption that increases anxiety about world events

Problematic Usage Patterns:

- **Compulsive checking**: Reaching for phone every few minutes throughout day

- **Sleep disruption**: Using devices until late night and checking upon waking

- **Mood dependency**: Emotional state determined by online interactions and feedback

- **Social comparison**: Constant comparison to curated images and lifestyles of others

Cyberbullying Experience: Aiden became a target after posting photos from a family vacation that classmates mocked:

Incident Details:

- Photos shared on Instagram showing family trip to national park

- Comments mocking his appearance, family dynamics, and interests

- Screenshots shared across multiple platforms and group chats

- Teachers and administrators unaware of online harassment

Impact on Mental Health:

- Immediate shame and humiliation following cyberbullying incident

- Withdrawal from in-person social activities and relationships

- Increased time online seeking validation and distraction
- Development of body image concerns and social anxiety

Family Dynamics and Digital Wellness: Aiden's parents struggle to understand and address his technology use:

Parental Concerns:

- "He's always on that phone—we can't get him to put it down"
- Worry that social media is "making him depressed"
- Frustration with their own limited understanding of online platforms
- Conflict over screen time limits and device restrictions

Family Assessment:

- Parents use devices heavily themselves, modeling constant connectivity
- No established family rules about device-free times or spaces
- Limited communication about online experiences and safety
- Punitive rather than collaborative approach to technology management

Digital Wellness Planning: The treatment team develops a family-based approach to improving Aiden's relationship with technology:

Individual Therapy Components:

- **Cognitive-behavioral techniques**: Identifying and challenging social comparison thoughts
- **Mindfulness training**: Developing awareness of technology use triggers and emotions
- **Social skills development**: Building confidence for in-person interactions
- **Coping skills**: Healthy alternatives to social media for mood regulation

Family Therapy Elements:

- **Digital wellness education**: Understanding healthy technology use for all family members

- **Communication skills**: Improving discussions about online experiences

- **Boundary setting**: Collaborative development of family technology agreements

- **Modeling**: Parents examining and modifying their own device use patterns

School Collaboration: The treatment team works with Aiden's school to address cyberbullying and promote digital citizenship:

School-Based Interventions:

- **Cyberbullying response**: Involving school counselors and administrators in addressing online harassment

- **Digital citizenship curriculum**: Teaching students about responsible technology use

- **Peer support programs**: Connecting Aiden with trained peer mentors

- **Mental health resources**: Providing on-site counseling and support services

Social Media Literacy Development: Aiden learns critical thinking skills for navigating online environments:

Content Analysis Skills:

- Understanding how social media algorithms influence what content appears

- Recognizing manipulated images and unrealistic lifestyle portrayals

- Identifying commercial motivation behind influencer content

- Developing healthy skepticism about online information

Privacy and Safety Education:

- Understanding privacy settings and their limitations

- Learning to identify and report cyberbullying and harassment

- Developing strategies for positive online community participation

- Building awareness of digital footprint and long-term consequences

Healthy Technology Use Strategies: The family implements evidence-based approaches to technology management:

Environmental Modifications:

- **Device-free bedrooms**: Charging stations outside sleeping areas for all family members

- **Meal time boundaries**: No devices during family meals

- **Homework zones**: Designated technology-free study spaces

- **Family activity time**: Regular screen-free activities and outings

Mindful Usage Practices:

- **Intentional checking**: Scheduled times for social media use rather than constant access

- **Purpose identification**: Asking "What am I hoping to get from this?" before opening apps

- **Time awareness**: Using built-in screen time tracking to increase consciousness of usage

- **Alternative activities**: Developing non-digital hobbies and interests

Social Connection Building:

- **In-person activities**: Encouraging face-to-face social interactions and activities

- **Community involvement**: Participating in clubs, sports, or volunteer opportunities

- **Family bonding**: Regular one-on-one time with parents without devices

- **Peer support**: Facilitating friendships based on shared interests rather than online status

Six-Month Outcomes: Aiden shows significant improvement across multiple areas:

Mental Health Improvement:

- PHQ-A depression score decreased from 16 to 8

- Reduced anxiety about social situations and peer interactions

- Improved sleep quality with consistent bedtime routine

- Increased self-esteem and body image acceptance

Technology Relationship:

- Decreased daily screen time from 8 hours to 3-4 hours

- More intentional and mindful technology use

- Reduced emotional reactivity to social media content

- Increased engagement in offline activities and relationships

Family Functioning:

- Improved communication about technology and online experiences

- Successful implementation of family digital wellness agreements

- Reduced conflict over device use and screen time

- Better modeling of healthy technology use by parents

Academic and Social Progress:

- Improved academic performance with better focus and study habits

- Increased participation in school activities and clubs

- Development of in-person friendships based on shared interests

- Leadership role in school's digital citizenship program

Case Study 11.3: Post-Pandemic Healthcare Worker Burnout

Jennifer Martinez, a 38-year-old ICU nurse with 15 years of experience, presents with symptoms that have worsened significantly since the COVID-19 pandemic began. She describes feeling "empty inside" despite previously finding deep meaning in her nursing work and reports using alcohol daily to "numb the pain" of what she's witnessed.

Pandemic-Related Trauma Exposure: Jennifer's experience reflects widespread mental health impacts on healthcare workers during the pandemic (33, 34):

Direct Trauma Exposure:

- Witnessing unprecedented numbers of patient deaths

- Making triage decisions about scarce resources

- Working with inadequate personal protective equipment

- Exposure to colleagues' illnesses and deaths

Moral Injury:

- Unable to provide usual quality of care due to resource limitations
- Conflict between professional values and institutional constraints
- Guilt about patient outcomes beyond her control
- Feeling responsible for potential disease transmission to family

Chronic Stress:

- Extended work hours due to staffing shortages
- Constant fear of infection for self and family
- Rapidly changing protocols and treatment guidelines
- Media attention and public criticism of healthcare system

PTSD Symptom Development: Jennifer meets criteria for PTSD based on her pandemic experiences:

Re-experiencing Symptoms:

- Intrusive memories of patient deaths and suffering
- Nightmares about work situations and patient care
- Flashbacks triggered by hospital sounds or medical equipment
- Physical reactions to reminders of pandemic experiences

Avoidance Behaviors:

- Avoiding news coverage about COVID-19 or healthcare
- Reluctance to discuss work experiences with family or friends
- Decreased interest in professional development or nursing organizations
- Considering career change to avoid healthcare environments

Negative Cognitions and Mood:

- Beliefs about personal inadequacy as a nurse
- Guilt about surviving when patients died

- Loss of meaning and purpose in nursing work

- Emotional numbing and disconnection from others

Hyperarousal Symptoms:

- Difficulty sleeping despite exhaustion

- Increased startle response and hypervigilance

- Irritability and anger outbursts

- Difficulty concentrating on tasks

Substance Use Development: Jennifer's alcohol use began as stress relief but has become problematic:

Progression Pattern:

- Started with occasional wine after difficult shifts

- Increased to daily drinking during pandemic peak

- Using alcohol to fall asleep and manage anxiety

- Drinking before work to cope with anticipatory anxiety

Functional Impact:

- Calling in sick more frequently

- Decreased job performance and medication errors

- Relationship conflicts with husband and children

- Physical health problems including sleep disruption and gastrointestinal issues

Peer Support Integration: Jennifer participates in a healthcare worker support group specifically designed for pandemic-related trauma:

Group Characteristics:

- **Membership**: ICU nurses, respiratory therapists, and physicians from local hospitals

- **Leadership**: Co-facilitated by mental health professional and experienced nurse

- **Format**: Weekly 90-minute sessions combining education and process work

- **Focus**: Moral injury, trauma processing, and professional identity restoration

Group Process Benefits:

- **Validation**: Hearing similar experiences from trusted colleagues
- **Normalization**: Understanding that distressing reactions are normal responses to abnormal situations
- **Skill sharing**: Learning coping strategies from other healthcare workers
- **Professional identity**: Reconnecting with values and meaning in healthcare work

Moral Injury Processing: The group addresses moral injury—psychological damage from perpetrating, witnessing, or failing to prevent acts that violate moral beliefs:

Moral Injury Themes:

- Being unable to provide comfort to dying patients due to isolation protocols
- Rationing care and making decisions about resource allocation
- Feeling complicit in a healthcare system that prioritized profits over patient care
- Guilt about being healthy while patients suffered and died

Healing Approaches:

- **Meaning-making**: Finding purpose and significance in pandemic service
- **Self-compassion**: Developing kindness toward self for doing the best possible under impossible circumstances
- **Values clarification**: Reconnecting with core nursing values and professional identity
- **Advocacy**: Channeling moral distress into efforts to improve healthcare systems

Organizational Response and Systemic Interventions: Jennifer's hospital implements system-level changes to address healthcare worker mental health:

Immediate Support Measures:

- **Employee assistance program**: Expanded mental health benefits and crisis counseling
- **Peer support teams**: Trained staff to provide immediate support after difficult cases

- **Wellness rooms**: Quiet spaces for rest and emotional regulation during shifts

- **Chaplain services**: Spiritual care for staff regardless of religious affiliation

Long-term System Changes:

- **Staffing improvements**: Hiring additional nurses to reduce workload and overtime

- **Safety protocols**: Better personal protective equipment and infection control measures

- **Communication enhancement**: Regular updates and transparency about institutional decisions

- **Professional development**: Supporting continuing education and career advancement

Leadership Training:

- **Trauma-informed management**: Teaching supervisors to recognize and respond to trauma symptoms

- **Mental health literacy**: Educating managers about mental health resources and referral processes

- **Resilience building**: Implementing evidence-based resilience training programs

- **Workload management**: Strategies for preventing burnout and promoting sustainable practice

Treatment Outcomes: After six months of integrated treatment, Jennifer shows significant improvement:

PTSD Symptom Reduction:

- Decreased frequency and intensity of intrusive memories

- Improved sleep quality with trauma-focused therapy

- Reduced avoidance of work-related activities and discussions

- Better emotional regulation and decreased hyperarousal

Substance Use Recovery:

- Achieved sobriety with combination of medical support and peer accountability

- Developed healthy coping strategies for work stress

- Improved physical health and energy levels

- Strengthened relationships with family members

Professional Re-engagement:

- Returns to full-time ICU nursing with renewed sense of purpose

- Takes leadership role in hospital's wellness committee

- Mentors new nurses and provides peer support to colleagues

- Advocates for systemic changes to support healthcare worker mental health

Jennifer's Reflection: "I thought I was broken—that I couldn't be a good nurse anymore after everything we went through. But I learned that my reactions were normal responses to an abnormal situation. Getting help didn't make me weak; it made me a better nurse and a better person."

Addressing Contemporary Mental Health Challenges

These three cases illustrate how emerging mental health challenges require adaptation of traditional therapeutic approaches while maintaining core principles of psychiatric nursing:

Environmental Health Connection: Climate anxiety represents a new category of anxiety disorder requiring validation of legitimate concerns while building psychological resilience for long-term environmental advocacy.

Technology and Mental Health Interface: Social media-related mental health problems require understanding of digital environments and development of digital wellness skills for both patients and families.

Systemic Trauma Response: Healthcare worker burnout and moral injury require both individual treatment and organizational interventions to address systemic causes of distress.

Nursing Competencies for Emerging Challenges:

- **Current events awareness**: Understanding how social and environmental issues affect mental health

- **Technology literacy**: Knowledge of digital platforms and their psychological impacts

- **Systems thinking**: Recognizing how organizational and societal factors contribute to individual distress

- **Advocacy skills**: Ability to address systemic causes of mental health problems

- **Cultural competence**: Understanding how emerging challenges affect different populations differently

Connection to Complex Cases

The skills developed for addressing emerging mental health challenges prepare you for managing complex multi-system cases that involve legal, cultural, and social factors. These contemporary issues often intersect with traditional psychiatric conditions in ways that require sophisticated clinical reasoning and interprofessional collaboration.

The next chapter examines complex cases that challenge you to integrate all the skills developed throughout this textbook while managing multiple systems and stakeholders.

Emerging Challenge Insights

- Climate anxiety requires validation of legitimate environmental concerns while building psychological resilience

- Social media-related mental health problems need both individual therapy and family-based digital wellness planning

- Healthcare worker burnout demands both individual treatment and organizational system changes

- Meaning-focused therapy helps patients maintain important commitments while developing sustainable practices

- Peer support groups provide unique benefits for people with shared professional or environmental experiences

- Technology literacy is essential for understanding and addressing digital mental health challenges

- Advocacy skills help nurses address systemic causes of emerging mental health problems

- Contemporary challenges often require both traditional therapeutic approaches and innovative interventions

Chapter 12: Complex Multi-System Cases

The phone call comes at 2:47 AM. A 17-year-old transgender youth sits in the emergency department after a suicide attempt, rejected by family, homeless, and facing criminal charges for defending themselves against assault. The case involves child protective services, juvenile court, LGBTQ+ advocacy organizations, and a complex web of medical, psychiatric, legal, and social systems that must work together—or watch a young person fall through the cracks.

Complex cases like this one demand every skill you've developed as a psychiatric nurse while pushing you into unfamiliar territory where clinical expertise intersects with legal requirements, cultural sensitivity, and ethical dilemmas. You become a translator between systems, an advocate for patients who can't advocate for themselves, and a coordinator of care that spans multiple agencies and jurisdictions.

Case Study 12.1: Forensic Psychiatric Scenario

Marcus Thompson, a 26-year-old man with antisocial personality disorder, stands trial for armed robbery. The court orders a competency evaluation to determine if he can understand the charges against him and assist in his own defense. Your role as the forensic psychiatric nurse involves assessing his mental state while navigating the complex intersection of mental health care and the criminal justice system.

Legal Framework for Competency Evaluation: The legal system requires defendants to be mentally competent to stand trial, based on established criteria:

Competency Standards:

- **Understanding of charges**: Can the defendant comprehend the nature and severity of accusations against them?

- **Understanding of proceedings**: Do they grasp the roles of judge, jury, prosecutor, and defense attorney?

- **Ability to assist counsel**: Can they communicate rationally with their attorney and participate in their defense?

- **Rational decision-making**: Are they capable of making informed decisions about plea bargains or trial strategy?

Assessment Challenges with Antisocial Personality Disorder: Marcus's personality disorder complicates the evaluation process:

Diagnostic Considerations:

- **Manipulation and deception**: Marcus may exaggerate symptoms to avoid prosecution or minimize them to appear competent

- **Lack of genuine remorse**: His apparent indifference to victims' suffering doesn't necessarily indicate incompetence

- **Antisocial attitudes**: Disregard for authority and social norms doesn't equal inability to understand legal proceedings

- **Substance use history**: Past drug use may have caused cognitive impairment separate from personality disorder

Forensic Assessment Process: The evaluation requires multiple sessions and collateral information sources:

Clinical Interviews: Session 1: Marcus presents as calm and articulate, readily discussing his charges and legal situation. He demonstrates clear understanding of the robbery accusations and potential penalties. However, he shows no emotional response to discussing the victim's trauma.

Marcus: "I understand they're saying I robbed that store. I know I could get 5-10 years if convicted. My lawyer wants me to consider a plea deal."

Nurse: "How do you feel about the possibility of prison time?"

Marcus: "It's part of the game. You win some, you lose some. The old lady will get over it—she wasn't hurt that bad."

Session 2: Focused on Marcus's ability to work with his defense attorney and make rational decisions about his case.

Marcus: "My lawyer thinks the plea deal is good, but I think we can beat this at trial. The witnesses aren't that reliable, and the video footage is unclear."

Nurse: "Help me understand how you're weighing the risks and benefits of going to trial versus accepting the plea."

Marcus: "If I take the plea, I'm definitely going to prison for three years. If we go to trial, maybe I walk free, maybe I get the full ten years. I like those odds better than guaranteed prison time."

Collateral Information Gathering:

- **Legal records**: Previous arrests, convictions, and court-ordered evaluations
- **Medical records**: History of psychiatric treatment, substance abuse, and head injuries
- **Family interviews**: Information about childhood development and behavioral patterns
- **Attorney consultation**: Discussion of Marcus's participation in legal strategy development

Psychological Testing:

- **Cognitive assessment**: IQ testing to rule out intellectual disability
- **Personality assessment**: MMPI-2 and other instruments to evaluate psychological functioning
- **Malingering detection**: Tests designed to identify symptom exaggeration or fabrication
- **Competency-specific instruments**: Formal measures of trial competency understanding

Ethical Challenges in Forensic Practice: Working in forensic settings creates unique ethical dilemmas for psychiatric nurses:

Dual Loyalty Issues:

- **Patient vs. system**: Balancing Marcus's individual needs with court requirements
- **Confidentiality limitations**: Information gathered may be shared with legal system
- **Therapeutic vs. evaluative role**: Assessment for court differs from treatment provision
- **Advocacy boundaries**: Supporting patient rights while maintaining objectivity

Informed Consent Complexities: Marcus must understand that the evaluation is not confidential therapy:

- **Purpose explanation**: Clarifying that assessment is for court, not treatment
- **Confidentiality limits**: Information will be shared with attorneys and judge

- **Right to refuse**: Marcus can decline evaluation but faces legal consequences
- **Self-incrimination concerns**: Statements may be used against him in court

Professional Boundary Management:

- **Therapeutic relationship**: Building rapport for assessment without providing treatment
- **Objectivity maintenance**: Avoiding personal reactions to antisocial behaviors
- **Legal compliance**: Following court orders while maintaining nursing ethics
- **Documentation requirements**: Detailed records that may become legal evidence

Team Approach and Collaboration: Forensic cases require coordination among multiple professionals:

Evaluation Team:

- **Forensic psychiatrist**: Medical assessment and final competency determination
- **Forensic psychologist**: Psychological testing and cognitive evaluation
- **Psychiatric nurse**: Mental status assessment and behavioral observations
- **Social worker**: Collateral information gathering and family assessment

Legal System Interface:

- **Defense attorney**: Represents Marcus's interests and reviews evaluation findings
- **Prosecutor**: May request independent evaluation if disagreeing with findings
- **Judge**: Makes final competency determination based on professional recommendations
- **Court personnel**: Manage scheduling and documentation requirements

Competency Findings and Recommendations: After extensive evaluation, the team reaches conclusions about Marcus's competency:

Competency Determination: Marcus demonstrates competency to stand trial based on:

- **Clear understanding**: Accurately describes charges, potential penalties, and court procedures

- **Rational communication**: Engages meaningfully with attorney about defense strategy

- **Decision-making capacity**: Weighs plea options rationally, even if others disagree with his choice

- **Factual knowledge**: Understands roles of court personnel and trial process

Personality Disorder vs. Incompetence: The evaluation distinguishes between antisocial traits and legal incompetence:

- **Moral understanding**: Marcus knows his actions were illegal, even if he doesn't feel remorse

- **Reality testing**: No evidence of delusions, hallucinations, or severe cognitive impairment

- **Rational thinking**: His decisions may be self-serving but are logically consistent

- **Legal awareness**: Understands consequences of his choices and legal proceedings

Court Testimony and Report: The psychiatric nurse contributes to court proceedings through formal report and potential testimony:

Report Elements:

- **Assessment methodology**: Detailed description of evaluation process and tools used

- **Clinical findings**: Mental status examination results and behavioral observations

- **Competency analysis**: Specific evaluation of legal competency criteria

- **Recommendations**: Clear opinion about fitness to proceed with trial

Testimony Preparation:

- **Expert qualification**: Education, training, and experience in forensic assessment

- **Opinion basis**: Explaining how clinical findings support competency conclusions

- **Cross-examination readiness**: Anticipating challenges to assessment methods and conclusions

- **Professional demeanor**: Maintaining objectivity and avoiding advocacy for either side

Treatment Recommendations: While Marcus is competent to stand trial, the evaluation identifies treatment needs:

Personality Disorder Management:

- **Skills training**: Impulse control and anger management programs

- **Substance abuse treatment**: Addressing underlying addiction issues

- **Cognitive-behavioral therapy**: Targeting criminal thinking patterns

- **Medication evaluation**: Considering treatment for comorbid conditions

Correctional Mental Health: If incarcerated, Marcus will need ongoing psychiatric care:

- **Mental health screening**: Regular assessment for depression, anxiety, or psychosis

- **Crisis intervention**: Suicide prevention and mental health emergency response

- **Programming participation**: Therapeutic communities and rehabilitation programs

- **Discharge planning**: Community mental health connections for eventual release

Case Study 12.2: Maternal Mental Health Crisis

Fatima Al-Rashid, a 29-year-old mother who gave birth three weeks ago, presents to the emergency department with her husband and mother-in-law after expressing beliefs that her newborn daughter is "evil" and must be "protected from demonic influences." This case involves postpartum psychosis, cultural considerations, infant safety concerns, and complex family dynamics.

Postpartum Psychosis Presentation: Fatima's symptoms developed rapidly over the past week and represent a psychiatric emergency:

Psychotic Symptoms:

- **Delusions**: Beliefs that her baby is possessed or evil

- **Hallucinations**: Hearing voices telling her to "save" the baby through harmful actions

- **Disorganized thinking**: Confusion about time, place, and recent events

- **Paranoid ideation**: Suspicion that hospital staff want to harm her or steal the baby

Mood Symptoms:

- **Agitation**: Restlessness and inability to remain calm

- **Mood lability**: Rapid shifts between euphoria and despair

- **Irritability**: Anger at family members and healthcare providers

- **Emotional intensity**: Extreme reactions to minor stimuli

Functional Impairment:

- **Infant care**: Unable to safely care for newborn due to delusional beliefs

- **Self-care**: Neglecting personal hygiene and nutrition

- **Sleep disruption**: Awake for extended periods "protecting" the baby

- **Social withdrawal**: Refusing visitors and avoiding family interactions

Cultural Considerations and Family Dynamics: Fatima's Pakistani cultural background significantly influences her presentation and treatment planning:

Cultural Factors:

- **Religious beliefs**: Islamic faith shapes understanding of mental health and spiritual influences

- **Family structure**: Extended family involvement in childbearing and child-rearing decisions

- **Gender roles**: Traditional expectations about motherhood and women's mental health

- **Stigma**: Mental illness may be viewed as spiritual weakness or family shame

Extended Family Involvement: Fatima's mother-in-law plays a crucial role in family decision-making:

Mother-in-law's perspective: "This is not mental illness—she is being tested by God. We need prayers and spiritual healing, not Western medicine."

Husband's conflict: "I want to respect my mother's wishes, but I'm scared Fatima might hurt herself or the baby. I don't know what to believe."

Cultural Bridge-Building: The treatment team involves a cultural liaison who helps navigate religious and cultural concerns:

Cultural Consultant Role:

- **Translation**: Explaining psychiatric concepts in culturally relevant terms

- **Mediation**: Facilitating discussions between family and medical team

- **Resource connection**: Linking family with culturally competent community supports

- **Education**: Helping family understand postpartum psychosis while respecting cultural beliefs

Imam Consultation: The hospital chaplain arranges for an imam to speak with the family:

Imam's guidance: "Islam teaches us that Allah provides healing through many means, including medicine. Seeking treatment for illness is not a lack of faith—it's using the tools God has given us."

Infant Safety Assessment and Intervention: Protecting the newborn requires immediate action while maintaining family relationships:

Safety Risk Factors:

- **Delusional content**: Beliefs about baby being evil or needing "protection"

- **Command hallucinations**: Voices instructing harmful actions toward infant

- **Impaired judgment**: Unable to assess baby's needs or safety appropriately

- **Behavioral unpredictability**: Rapid changes in mental state and actions

Immediate Safety Measures:

- **Constant supervision**: Family member or nurse always present when Fatima interacts with baby

- **Environmental safety**: Removal of potential weapons or harmful objects

- **Feeding support**: Ensuring baby receives adequate nutrition through bottle feeding

- **Medical evaluation**: Pediatric assessment to ensure infant's physical health

Child Protective Services Involvement: The team involves CPS while working to keep the family together:

CPS Assessment:

- **Safety plan development**: Creating structure for safe infant care during mother's treatment

- **Family support evaluation**: Assessing extended family's ability to provide protection

- **Service coordination**: Connecting family with ongoing support and monitoring

- **Legal requirements**: Meeting mandatory reporting obligations while supporting family unity

Safety Plan Elements:

- **24-hour supervision**: Competent adult always present when mother and baby are together

- **Medication compliance**: Ensuring Fatima takes prescribed psychiatric medications

- **Follow-up appointments**: Regular mental health and pediatric visits

- **Emergency contacts**: Clear plan for crisis situations and immediate help

Treatment Planning with Cultural Integration: The team develops a treatment approach that respects cultural values while ensuring safety:

Medication Management:

- **Antipsychotic medication**: Rapid-acting medication to reduce psychotic symptoms

- **Cultural education**: Explaining medication necessity while respecting religious concerns

- **Breastfeeding considerations**: Discussing medication effects on nursing and infant

- **Family involvement**: Including husband and mother-in-law in medication education

Therapeutic Interventions:

- **Individual therapy**: Processing childbirth experience and adjusting to motherhood

- **Family therapy**: Addressing cultural conflicts and communication patterns

- **Postpartum support group**: Connecting with other mothers experiencing mental health challenges

- **Cultural therapy**: Working with culturally competent therapist familiar with Pakistani traditions

Spiritual Integration:

- **Prayer accommodation**: Providing space and time for religious observances

- **Imam counseling**: Regular spiritual guidance that supports mental health treatment

- **Religious community**: Connecting with mosque members who understand mental health

- **Faith-based coping**: Incorporating religious practices into recovery plan

Progress and Resolution: Fatima shows significant improvement with culturally sensitive treatment:

Week 1: Antipsychotic medication reduces hallucinations and delusions significantly

- Family begins to understand postpartum psychosis as medical condition

- Safety plan allows supervised interaction with baby

- Cultural liaison helps address religious concerns about medication

Week 3: Psychotic symptoms largely resolved, mood stabilizing

- Increased insight into illness and need for treatment

- Improved infant care abilities with continued supervision

- Family relationships strengthening with education and support

Month 2: Successful transition to outpatient care

- Independent infant care restored with family support system

- Regular follow-up with culturally competent psychiatrist

- Active participation in postpartum support group

- Integration of religious practices with mental health care

Six-Month Outcome: Full recovery with strong family bonds

- No recurrence of psychotic symptoms with medication maintenance

- Excellent mother-infant attachment and bonding

- Extended family supportive of mental health treatment

- Plans for future pregnancies include mental health monitoring

Case Study 12.3: Transgender Youth in Crisis

Alex Chen, a 17-year-old transgender male, presents to the emergency department following a serious suicide attempt. He was rejected by his family after coming out as transgender six months ago and has been living on the streets. Recent assault charges stem from defending himself against a transphobic attack, adding legal complications to his mental health crisis.

Complex Presentation Factors: Alex's case illustrates how multiple marginalized identities create compounding stressors:

Identity Development:

- **Gender dysphoria**: Persistent discomfort with birth-assigned female gender
- **Social transition**: Using male name and pronouns for the past year
- **Medical transition desires**: Wants hormone therapy and eventual surgical options
- **Family rejection**: Parents refuse to accept transgender identity

Trauma History:

- **Family rejection**: Emotional abuse and abandonment following disclosure
- **Homelessness**: Living on streets with exposure to violence and exploitation
- **Assault experience**: Recent physical attack motivated by anti-transgender bias
- **Systemic discrimination**: Difficulty accessing services due to transgender status

Legal Complications:

- **Assault charges**: Facing criminal charges for defending himself during attack
- **Age considerations**: Minor status complicates legal and medical decision-making
- **Documentation issues**: Legal name and gender markers don't match identity
- **Emancipation needs**: Seeking legal independence from rejecting parents

Mental Health Assessment: Alex presents with multiple psychiatric symptoms requiring immediate attention:

Suicide Risk Factors:

133

- **Recent attempt**: Serious overdose requiring medical intervention

- **High intent**: Clear plan and expectation of death

- **Multiple stressors**: Homelessness, family rejection, legal problems

- **Minority stress**: Discrimination and marginalization specific to transgender identity

Depression Symptoms:

- **Hopelessness**: "Nothing will ever get better for someone like me"

- **Worthlessness**: Internalized messages about transgender identity being "wrong"

- **Social isolation**: Limited support systems and safe relationships

- **Functional impairment**: Unable to attend school or maintain employment

Trauma Symptoms:

- **Hypervigilance**: Constant scanning for threats and dangers

- **Intrusive memories**: Flashbacks to assault and family rejection experiences

- **Avoidance**: Staying away from places and people that trigger trauma memories

- **Emotional numbing**: Disconnection from feelings as protection mechanism

Gender-Affirming Care Implementation: The treatment team implements evidence-based approaches for transgender youth mental health:

Affirming Environment Creation:

- **Name and pronouns**: Consistent use of Alex's chosen name and male pronouns

- **Room assignment**: Placement that respects gender identity and ensures safety

- **Staff education**: Training on transgender terminology and respectful care

- **Privacy protection**: Confidentiality regarding transgender status and medical information

Medical Care Coordination:

- **Hormone therapy evaluation**: Assessment for testosterone treatment readiness

- **Primary care needs**: Addressing general health concerns and preventive care

- **Mental health clearance**: Evaluation for gender-affirming medical treatments

- **Documentation support**: Assistance with legal name and gender marker changes

Safety Planning:

- **Immediate safety**: Secure, affirming placement during mental health stabilization

- **Long-term housing**: Connecting with LGBTQ+-affirming housing programs

- **Support systems**: Building relationships with affirming adults and peers

- **Crisis resources**: Access to transgender-specific crisis intervention services

Resource Coordination and System Navigation: Alex's care requires coordination across multiple systems and organizations:

LGBTQ+ Community Services:

- **Youth shelter**: Temporary housing specifically for LGBTQ+ homeless youth

- **Support groups**: Peer connections with other transgender young people

- **Advocacy organizations**: Legal support and resource navigation assistance

- **Community center**: Safe space for social connection and support services

Legal Support Systems:

- **LGBTQ+ legal clinic**: Pro bono legal representation for assault charges

- **Emancipation assistance**: Help with legal independence from parents

- **Name change support**: Legal process for updating identity documents

- **Educational advocacy**: Ensuring school access and anti-discrimination protection

Healthcare Navigation:

- **Transgender health clinic**: Specialized medical care for gender transition

- **Mental health services**: Therapists with expertise in transgender youth care

- **Insurance advocacy**: Assistance with coverage for gender-affirming treatments

- **Preventive care**: Ensuring access to routine healthcare and screening

Family Work and Relationship Healing: While Alex's parents are currently rejecting, the team explores possibilities for family reconciliation:

Family Assessment:

- **Cultural factors**: Chinese-American family dynamics and traditional gender expectations

- **Religious influences**: Impact of religious beliefs on acceptance of transgender identity

- **Educational needs**: Parents' understanding of transgender identity and medical care

- **Motivation evaluation**: Willingness to learn and potentially rebuild relationship

Family Intervention Approaches:

- **Educational resources**: Providing information about transgender identity and health

- **Support groups**: Connecting parents with other families of transgender youth

- **Cultural mediation**: Working with culturally competent family therapists

- **Gradual engagement**: Starting with minimal contact and building slowly if possible

Treatment Outcomes and Long-term Planning: Alex's recovery involves both immediate stabilization and long-term development planning:

Mental Health Stabilization:

- **Depression treatment**: Combination of medication and affirming therapy

- **Trauma processing**: Specialized therapy for assault and rejection experiences

- **Suicide risk reduction**: Safety planning and crisis prevention strategies

- **Identity development**: Support for healthy transgender identity formation

Social Support Building:

- **Peer connections**: Relationships with other transgender youth and allies

- **Mentor relationships**: Connections with affirming adults and role models

- **Community involvement**: Participation in LGBTQ+ advocacy and support activities

- **Educational re-engagement**: Return to school with appropriate support and protection

Future Planning:

- **Medical transition**: Continued gender-affirming medical care as appropriate

- **Educational goals**: College preparation and career planning

- **Independent living**: Skills development for successful adult independence

- **Advocacy involvement**: Potential leadership roles in LGBTQ+ community organizations

One-Year Outcome: Alex demonstrates remarkable resilience and recovery:

- Stable housing in affirming foster family placement

- Successful completion of high school with college acceptance

- No recurrence of suicidal ideation with ongoing mental health support

- Leadership role in local LGBTQ+ youth advocacy organization

- Limited but improving contact with parents through family therapy

Managing Complex Multi-System Cases

These three cases demonstrate the sophistication required for managing complex psychiatric situations that involve multiple systems, stakeholders, and competing interests:

Systems Coordination Skills:

- **Communication**: Facilitating understanding between different professional languages and priorities

- **Advocacy**: Representing patient interests while working within system constraints

- **Conflict resolution**: Managing disagreements between systems and stakeholders

- **Resource navigation**: Connecting patients with appropriate services across multiple agencies

Cultural and Legal Competence:

- **Cultural humility**: Adapting interventions to respect diverse values and beliefs

- **Legal awareness**: Understanding how laws affect patient care and treatment options

- **Ethical reasoning**: Balancing competing obligations and interests

- **Boundary management**: Maintaining professional roles while addressing complex needs

Professional Development Requirements:

- **Interdisciplinary collaboration**: Working effectively with legal, social service, and community professionals

- **Specialized knowledge**: Understanding forensic, perinatal, and LGBTQ+ health issues

- **Crisis management**: Responding effectively to emergencies while coordinating multiple systems

- **Long-term planning**: Developing sustainable solutions that address root causes of problems

Looking Toward Professional Excellence

The complex cases in this chapter represent the most challenging scenarios you'll encounter as a psychiatric nurse. They require integration of all the skills developed throughout this textbook while pushing you to grow professionally and personally.

These cases also illustrate why psychiatric nursing remains fundamentally about human relationships—even when legal systems, cultural differences, and social challenges complicate the clinical picture, your ability to connect authentically with patients and advocate for their wellbeing makes the difference between recovery and continued suffering.

Complex Case Management Foundations

- Multi-system cases require coordination across legal, social service, healthcare, and community organizations

- Cultural competence must be maintained even when cultural values conflict with clinical recommendations

- Patient safety remains the priority while respecting autonomy and cultural values

- Forensic nursing requires understanding legal frameworks and maintaining objectivity

- Maternal mental health cases need rapid intervention while preserving family relationships

- LGBTQ+ youth require affirming care and specialized resources for optimal outcomes

- Professional boundaries become more complex when multiple systems are involved

- Advocacy skills are essential for representing patient interests across different systems

Closing Perspective

These complex multi-system cases represent the most challenging and rewarding aspects of psychiatric nursing practice. They require you to function as clinician, advocate, educator, and coordinator while maintaining the therapeutic relationships that remain at the heart of healing.

The cases presented throughout this textbook—from basic assessment skills to complex forensic scenarios—prepare you for the full spectrum of psychiatric nursing practice. Each patient you encounter will teach you something new about human resilience, the power of therapeutic relationships, and your own capacity to make a difference in people's lives.

Your willingness to engage with these complex challenges, to advocate for vulnerable populations, and to continue learning throughout your career will determine not only your success as a psychiatric nurse but also your contribution to the profession's ongoing development. The patients who trust you with their most vulnerable moments deserve nothing less than your best effort to provide competent, compassionate, evidence-based care.

Chapter 13: Crisis Intervention and Disaster Response

The crisis call arrives at 3:17 AM on a Tuesday—a woman threatening to jump from a downtown bridge while traffic backs up for miles in both directions. Your mobile crisis team loads into the van with equipment, protocols, and years of training, but you know the most important tools you carry are your voice, your presence, and your ability to connect with someone in their darkest moment.

Crisis intervention represents psychiatric nursing at its most immediate and high-stakes. There's no time for lengthy assessments or gradual rapport building. You must quickly establish trust, assess safety, and implement interventions that can mean the difference between life and death. These skills serve you whether you're responding to community emergencies, natural disasters, or the daily crises that unfold in hospitals and clinics.

Mobile Crisis Team Scenarios

Community-based crisis intervention has revolutionized how mental health emergencies are managed. Instead of relying solely on police response or emergency department visits, mobile crisis teams bring mental health expertise directly to people experiencing psychiatric emergencies in their homes, schools, workplaces, and community settings.

Crisis Response Case Study 13.1: Domestic Violence and Suicide Risk

The call comes through dispatch at 11:30 PM: "Female, age 32, threatening suicide after domestic violence incident. Police on scene, requesting mental health response." Sarah, the mobile crisis nurse, and Jim, the crisis counselor, arrive at a small apartment complex where police cars block the parking lot and neighbors peer from windows.

Scene Assessment and Safety: Mobile crisis teams must rapidly assess multiple levels of safety before engaging with clients:

Environmental Safety:

- **Police presence**: Officers have secured the scene and separated the domestic violence perpetrator

- **Bystander management**: Neighbors are curious but not threatening the situation

- **Physical hazards**: Broken glass and overturned furniture from the altercation

- **Escape routes**: Clear pathways identified in case rapid evacuation becomes necessary

Client Safety:

- **Immediate medical needs**: Lisa has visible bruises but refuses ambulance transport

- **Suicide risk factors**: Has taken an unknown number of pills and made explicit threats

- **Weapon access**: No weapons visible, but kitchen knives are accessible

- **Intoxication level**: Appears sober despite pill ingestion

Team Safety:

- **Communication**: Constant radio contact with dispatch and police backup

- **Positioning**: Maintaining safe distance while building rapport

- **Equipment**: Emergency medications and crisis intervention supplies available

- **Exit strategy**: Clear plan for immediate withdrawal if situation deteriorates

Initial Engagement and Rapport Building: Lisa sits on her couch, arms wrapped around herself, refusing to make eye contact with anyone. Her 8-year-old daughter sleeps in the bedroom, apparently unaware of the crisis unfolding.

Sarah's Approach: "Hi Lisa, I'm Sarah, a nurse with the crisis team. I can see you've had a really difficult night. Can you help me understand what's happening right now?"

Lisa (barely audible): "I just want everyone to leave me alone. I can't do this anymore."

Sarah: "It sounds like you're feeling overwhelmed and exhausted. That makes sense after what you've been through. I'm here to listen and help figure out what needs to happen next."

Lisa: "Nothing needs to happen. I've already decided what I'm going to do."

Crisis Assessment Protocol: The mobile team follows a structured assessment process while maintaining therapeutic engagement:

Suicide Risk Assessment:

- **Ideation**: "I keep thinking about taking the rest of the pills"

- **Plan**: Has access to remaining medication, knows lethal dose from internet research

- **Intent**: "I'm tired of being hurt and disappointing everyone"

- **Means**: Multiple prescription bottles accessible
- **Timeline**: "Maybe after my daughter goes to school tomorrow"

Protective Factors:

- **Daughter**: Strong maternal attachment and responsibility
- **Support system**: Sister who lives nearby and has helped before
- **Previous coping**: Successfully left abusive relationship once before
- **Treatment history**: Positive experience with counseling two years ago

Safety Planning: Sarah works with Lisa to develop immediate safety strategies:

Immediate Interventions:

- **Medication securing**: Police will temporarily hold all medications
- **Support activation**: Sister contacted and agrees to stay overnight
- **Child care planning**: Daughter can stay with sister if needed
- **Crisis contacts**: Mobile team and crisis hotline numbers provided

24-Hour Plan:

- **Medical evaluation**: Agreement to see family doctor about injuries and medication concerns
- **Counseling appointment**: Crisis team will arrange therapy session within 48 hours
- **Legal consultation**: Information provided about domestic violence legal protections
- **Follow-up contact**: Crisis team will call tomorrow evening

Community Resource Coordination: The team coordinates multiple services to address Lisa's complex needs:

Domestic Violence Services:

- **Shelter information**: Safe housing options if she chooses to leave permanently
- **Legal advocacy**: Assistance with restraining orders and court proceedings
- **Safety planning**: Strategies for protection if she remains in current housing

- **Support groups**: Connections with other domestic violence survivors

Child Welfare Considerations:

- **Safety assessment**: Ensuring daughter's immediate and ongoing protection
- **School notification**: Alerting school counselors about family crisis
- **Support services**: Counseling resources for children exposed to domestic violence
- **Family preservation**: Working to keep family together safely

Mental Health Services:

- **Emergency psychiatry**: Medication evaluation and crisis stabilization
- **Ongoing therapy**: Individual counseling for trauma and relationship issues
- **Case management**: Coordination of multiple services and follow-up care
- **Support groups**: Peer support for depression and domestic violence survivors

Outcome and Follow-up: Lisa agrees to safety plan and accepts voluntary services rather than requiring involuntary commitment. Three-month follow-up shows significant improvement: she's engaged in therapy, obtained restraining order, and reports no suicidal ideation. Her daughter receives counseling and shows resilience with appropriate support.

Crisis Response Case Study 13.2: Adolescent School Crisis

The high school principal calls the mobile crisis team after 16-year-old Marcus is found in the bathroom with self-inflicted cuts on his arms. He's refusing to speak with school counselors and threatens to "finish the job" if his parents are contacted. The situation requires delicate balance between adolescent autonomy, safety concerns, and legal requirements.

School-Based Crisis Intervention: Educational settings present unique challenges for crisis response:

Confidentiality Considerations:

- **FERPA requirements**: Educational privacy laws affecting information sharing
- **Parental notification**: Balancing adolescent privacy with parental rights
- **Mandatory reporting**: School obligations for child welfare reporting

- **Peer confidentiality**: Preventing rumors and protecting student privacy

Environmental Management:

- **Location privacy**: Moving Marcus to nurse's office away from other students

- **Crowd control**: Keeping curious students and staff away from crisis area

- **Normal operations**: Maintaining school routine while addressing emergency

- **Media management**: Preventing news coverage or social media attention

Adolescent Engagement Strategies: Working with teenagers in crisis requires specialized approaches:

Development Considerations:

- **Identity formation**: Understanding adolescent identity development pressures

- **Peer influence**: Recognizing importance of social relationships and status

- **Authority relationships**: Adapting approach for adolescent resistance to adult authority

- **Future orientation**: Limited ability to see beyond current crisis

Marcus's Initial Response: "I'm not talking to any more adults. You all just make things worse."

Crisis Nurse Approach: "That sounds like adults have disappointed you before. I get why you might not trust another one. What would need to be different for you to feel like someone actually understood?"

Marcus: "Nobody gets what it's like to be me. Everyone expects me to be perfect, and I'm just... not."

Assessment in School Setting: The crisis team adapts assessment techniques for the school environment:

Risk Factor Identification:

- **Academic pressure**: Struggling with advanced placement classes and college expectations

- **Social isolation**: Recent friendship loss and bullying experiences

- **Family expectations**: High-achieving parents with limited understanding of mental health

- **Identity questions**: Confusion about sexual orientation and fear of family rejection

Self-Harm Behavior Analysis:

- **Cutting history**: Started six months ago as stress relief mechanism

- **Escalation pattern**: Frequency and severity increasing over past month

- **Function**: Uses cutting to "feel something" and manage emotional numbness

- **Concealment**: Careful to hide cuts and maintain appearance of functioning

School Resource Utilization:

- **Counseling services**: School psychologist available for ongoing support

- **Academic accommodations**: Possible modifications for mental health needs

- **Peer support**: Identification of positive peer relationships and mentors

- **Extracurricular engagement**: Activities that provide meaning and connection

Safety Planning for Adolescents: Adolescent safety planning requires age-appropriate approaches:

Collaborative Development: Marcus participates in creating his own safety plan rather than having one imposed:

Warning Signs Recognition:

- **Emotional**: Feeling "empty" or overwhelmed by expectations

- **Behavioral**: Isolating from friends, declining grades, sleep changes

- **Physical**: Increased urges to self-harm or thoughts of suicide

- **Social**: Conflicts with parents or teachers about performance

Coping Strategies:

- **Alternative behaviors**: Holding ice cubes, drawing on skin with red marker

- **Support activation**: Texting trusted friend, talking to school counselor

- **Environmental changes**: Removing or securing sharp objects

- **Self-care**: Exercise, music, time in nature

Support System Activation:

- **School contacts**: Counselor, trusted teacher, and peer mentor

- **Community resources**: LGBTQ+ youth center and crisis text line

- **Family involvement**: Gradual education and engagement of parents

- **Professional support**: Arrangement for ongoing therapy

Parent Engagement Strategy: The team carefully manages parental involvement to maintain Marcus's trust while ensuring family support:

Preparation Phase:

- **Marcus's input**: Discussion about what he wants parents to know

- **Educational approach**: Providing parents with information about adolescent mental health

- **Support for parents**: Resources for families dealing with mental health crises

- **Collaborative planning**: Including parents in safety planning and treatment decisions

Family Meeting Facilitation:

- **Safe environment**: Neutral location with crisis team present

- **Structured communication**: Guidelines for productive discussion

- **Education provision**: Information about self-harm, suicide risk, and treatment options

- **Ongoing support**: Referrals for family therapy and parent support groups

Mass Casualty Mental Health Response

Large-scale disasters create unique mental health challenges that require coordinated response from multiple agencies and organizations. Psychiatric nurses play critical roles in disaster mental health response, providing immediate crisis support and longer-term recovery services.

Disaster Response Case Study 13.3: Tornado Community Impact

A category F4 tornado strikes a rural community of 15,000 people, destroying 200 homes, damaging the high school and hospital, and killing 12 residents. The state activates disaster mental health response teams to provide immediate and ongoing psychological support to survivors, first responders, and community members.

Immediate Response Phase (0-72 hours):

Psychological First Aid Principles: Disaster mental health response follows evidence-based psychological first aid principles:

Contact and Engagement:

- **Proactive outreach**: Mental health teams move through shelters and affected neighborhoods
- **Non-intrusive approach**: Offering support without forcing interaction
- **Cultural sensitivity**: Understanding community values and communication styles
- **Practical assistance**: Helping with immediate needs while building trust

Safety and Comfort:

- **Physical safety**: Ensuring basic needs for food, shelter, and medical care are met
- **Emotional safety**: Creating calm environments and reducing additional stressors
- **Connection facilitation**: Helping people contact family and support systems
- **Information provision**: Accurate updates about rescue efforts and available resources

Stabilization:

- **Emotional regulation**: Teaching basic grounding and calming techniques
- **Information processing**: Helping people understand normal stress reactions
- **Coping activation**: Encouraging use of existing coping skills and resources
- **Hope instillation**: Focusing on survival, community support, and recovery possibilities

Community Response Coordination: Disaster mental health requires coordination among multiple agencies:

Response Team Composition:

- **Mental health professionals**: Psychiatrists, nurses, social workers, counselors
- **Peer support specialists**: Community members trained in disaster response
- **Chaplains**: Spiritual care providers from various faith traditions
- **Cultural liaisons**: Representatives from different cultural communities

Service Delivery Models:

- **Mobile teams**: Bringing services directly to affected areas
- **Shelter support**: Mental health presence in emergency shelters
- **Family assistance centers**: Centralized location for multiple services
- **Community meetings**: Group education and support sessions

Special Population Considerations: Different groups within the community require adapted approaches:

Children and Adolescents:

- **School-based services**: Mental health support in temporary educational settings
- **Family-centered approach**: Working with parents and caregivers to support children
- **Developmental considerations**: Age-appropriate explanations and interventions
- **Play therapy techniques**: Using art, games, and expressive activities

Older Adults:

- **Medical needs integration**: Coordinating mental health care with medical services
- **Medication management**: Ensuring continued access to psychiatric medications
- **Social support**: Addressing isolation and displacement issues
- **Cognitive considerations**: Adapting interventions for dementia or cognitive impairment

First Responders:

- **Stress debriefing**: Structured processing of traumatic experiences

- **Peer support programs**: Fellow first responders providing mutual support

- **Family services**: Supporting families of first responders

- **Return-to-duty assessment**: Evaluating readiness to resume emergency work

Long-term Recovery Phase (3 months - 2 years):

Community Recovery Services:

- **Outreach and case finding**: Identifying people needing ongoing mental health support

- **Treatment services**: Individual and group therapy for trauma and grief

- **Support groups**: Peer-led groups for different affected populations

- **Community education**: Training programs about trauma and resilience

Service Integration:

- **Primary care coordination**: Training medical providers in trauma screening

- **School-based programs**: Ongoing mental health services in educational settings

- **Workplace support**: Employee assistance programs for affected businesses

- **Faith community partnerships**: Working with religious organizations

Crisis Intervention Team Model

The Crisis Intervention Team (CIT) model represents best practices for police-mental health collaboration in responding to psychiatric emergencies. This approach reduces injuries, decreases arrests of people with mental illness, and improves connections to treatment services.

CIT Training Components:

Police Officer Education:

- **Mental illness awareness**: Understanding symptoms and behaviors of psychiatric conditions

- **De-escalation techniques**: Verbal and non-verbal strategies for reducing agitation

- **Legal considerations**: Understanding commitment laws and patient rights

- **Community resources**: Knowledge of available mental health services

Mental Health Professional Training:

- **Law enforcement culture**: Understanding police procedures and safety concerns

- **Crisis intervention**: Rapid assessment and intervention techniques

- **Safety awareness**: Managing personal safety during crisis responses

- **Legal requirements**: Documentation and testimony requirements

Collaborative Response Protocols:

- **Joint response teams**: Mental health professionals accompanying police to crisis calls

- **Consultation services**: Phone consultation for officers responding to mental health calls

- **Follow-up services**: Ensuring connection to ongoing mental health care

- **Quality improvement**: Regular review and improvement of response protocols

Simulation Exercises and Training

High-fidelity crisis simulation provides safe environments for practicing crisis intervention skills and testing response protocols.

Simulation Scenario Design:

Standardized Patients:

- **Realistic presentations**: Actors trained to portray specific psychiatric conditions

- **Consistent challenges**: Standardized scenarios for reliable training experiences

- **Safety considerations**: Protocols for managing intense emotional content

- **Feedback provision**: Structured debriefing about performance and learning

Environmental Realism:

- **Community settings**: Simulations in homes, schools, workplaces

- **Equipment availability**: Crisis intervention supplies and communication devices

- **Time pressure**: Realistic time constraints and urgency

- **Interprofessional teams**: Including police, paramedics, and social workers

Learning Objectives:

- **Assessment skills**: Rapid mental status evaluation and risk assessment
- **Communication techniques**: De-escalation and rapport building
- **Safety management**: Personal and client safety in crisis situations
- **Resource coordination**: Connecting clients with appropriate services

Debriefing and Improvement:

- **Performance review**: Video analysis and peer feedback
- **Skill development**: Identifying areas for improvement and additional training
- **Protocol refinement**: Using simulation results to improve response procedures
- **Confidence building**: Increasing comfort with crisis intervention skills

Professional Development in Crisis Services

Crisis intervention work requires ongoing professional development and support:

Specialized Training Requirements:

- **Crisis intervention certification**: Formal training programs and credentialing
- **Trauma-informed care**: Understanding trauma impacts and recovery principles
- **Cultural competence**: Working effectively with diverse populations
- **Legal and ethical issues**: Managing complex situations with legal implications

Self-Care and Burnout Prevention:

- **Stress management**: Personal strategies for managing high-stress work
- **Peer support**: Colleague relationships and mutual assistance
- **Professional consultation**: Regular supervision and case review
- **Work-life balance**: Maintaining personal health and relationships

Career Pathways:

- **Community mental health**: Outpatient crisis and intensive services

- **Emergency services**: Hospital-based crisis intervention

- **Disaster response**: Specialized training in mass casualty mental health

- **Program development**: Leadership roles in crisis service design and implementation

Building Crisis Response Competence

Crisis intervention represents one of the most challenging and rewarding areas of psychiatric nursing practice. The ability to help people during their most difficult moments requires both technical skills and personal qualities that develop over time.

Success in crisis work depends on your ability to remain calm under pressure, think clearly during chaos, and maintain hope when others have lost theirs. These skills transfer to all areas of nursing practice and make you a more effective clinician regardless of your specialty area.

The next chapter examines how quality improvement principles help crisis services and all psychiatric nursing programs continuously improve their effectiveness and outcomes.

Crisis Intervention Essentials

- Mobile crisis teams provide community-based alternatives to emergency department visits and police responses

- Safety assessment and management are fundamental to all crisis intervention activities

- Adolescent crisis intervention requires specialized approaches that respect developmental needs

- Disaster mental health response follows psychological first aid principles and requires coordinated community effort

- Crisis Intervention Team models improve police-mental health collaboration and outcomes

- Simulation training provides safe environments for developing and testing crisis intervention skills

- Professional development in crisis work requires ongoing training, supervision, and self-care practices

- Crisis intervention skills transfer to all areas of nursing practice and improve overall clinical effectiveness

Chapter 14: Quality Improvement and Evidence-Based Practice

The monthly unit meeting reveals troubling statistics: psychiatric readmission rates have increased by 15% over six months, patient satisfaction scores are declining, and staff turnover has reached an all-time high. As the nurse manager presents these numbers, you recognize that good intentions and hard work aren't enough—systematic approaches to quality improvement and evidence-based practice are necessary to provide the best possible care for patients and support for staff.

Quality improvement in psychiatric nursing requires you to think like both a clinician and a scientist. You must identify problems systematically, search for evidence-based solutions, implement changes thoughtfully, and measure outcomes rigorously. This process transforms nursing practice from tradition-based routines to data-driven excellence that continuously adapts to new knowledge and changing patient needs.

QI Project Development for Mental Health Units

Quality improvement projects in psychiatric settings address unique challenges related to patient safety, treatment effectiveness, staff competence, and regulatory compliance. Successful projects require clear problem identification, stakeholder engagement, evidence review, and systematic implementation.

QI Case Study 14.1: Reducing Psychiatric Readmissions

Metro General Hospital's 30-bed inpatient psychiatric unit faces a crisis: 30-day readmission rates have climbed to 28%, well above the national average of 20%. The hospital administration demands improvement, threatening to close the unit if rates don't decrease within six months. The nursing staff forms a quality improvement team to address this challenge.

Problem Identification and Root Cause Analysis:

Data Collection and Analysis: The QI team gathers comprehensive data to understand readmission patterns:

Quantitative Measures:

- **Readmission timing**: 65% of readmissions occur within 14 days of discharge

- **Diagnosis patterns**: Patients with bipolar disorder and schizophrenia have highest readmission rates

- **Demographic factors**: Younger patients and those with co-occurring substance use show increased risk

- **Length of stay**: Patients with shorter initial stays (less than 5 days) readmit more frequently

Qualitative Assessment:

- **Patient interviews**: Exit interviews reveal confusion about medications and follow-up appointments

- **Family feedback**: Families report feeling unprepared to support patients at home

- **Staff observations**: Discharge planning often rushed due to bed pressure

- **Community provider input**: Outpatient providers report poor communication about treatment plans

Root Cause Analysis Findings: Using fishbone diagram analysis, the team identifies primary contributing factors:

Process Issues:

- **Discharge planning**: Started too late in admission, often day of discharge

- **Medication education**: Limited time allocated, focus on compliance rather than understanding

- **Follow-up coordination**: Appointments scheduled but not confirmed with patients

- **Communication gaps**: Poor information transfer between inpatient and outpatient providers

Resource Constraints:

- **Staffing**: High patient-to-nurse ratios limiting individual attention

- **Time pressure**: Average length of stay decreased due to insurance pressure

- **Community resources**: Limited availability of immediate outpatient appointments

- **Transportation**: Many patients lack reliable transportation to follow-up appointments

System Factors:

- **Bed management**: Pressure to discharge quickly for new admissions

- **Insurance authorization**: Coverage limitations affecting treatment options

- **Community coordination**: Limited relationships with outpatient providers

- **Crisis services**: Inadequate community crisis support leading to readmissions

Evidence Review and Best Practices: The team conducts literature review to identify evidence-based strategies for reducing psychiatric readmissions:

Transition Care Models:

- **Bridge programs**: Intensive outpatient services immediately following discharge

- **Peer support**: Trained peers providing support during transition period

- **Case management**: Dedicated staff coordinating services and monitoring progress

- **Telehealth follow-up**: Technology-enabled monitoring and support

Medication Management:

- **Medication reconciliation**: Systematic review of all medications at discharge

- **Simplified regimens**: Reducing pill burden and dosing frequency when possible

- **Injectable medications**: Long-acting formulations for patients with adherence challenges

- **Pharmacy coordination**: Direct communication between hospital and community pharmacies

Family Engagement:

- **Education programs**: Structured teaching about mental illness and recovery

- **Support groups**: Ongoing support for families and caregivers

- **Communication training**: Teaching families how to communicate with patients about mental health

- **Crisis planning**: Involving families in safety planning and crisis prevention

Intervention Design and Implementation:

SMART Goals Development: The team establishes specific, measurable, achievable, relevant, and time-bound goals:

Primary Goal: Reduce 30-day psychiatric readmission rates from 28% to 18% within six months

Secondary Goals:

- Increase follow-up appointment attendance from 60% to 80%

- Improve patient satisfaction with discharge planning from 3.2 to 4.0 (5-point scale)

- Decrease average time from admission to discharge planning initiation from 3 days to 1 day

Intervention Bundle Implementation: The team implements multiple evidence-based interventions simultaneously:

Enhanced Discharge Planning Process:

- **Day-one planning**: Discharge planning begins within 24 hours of admission

- **Multidisciplinary rounds**: Daily team meetings including patient and family

- **Standardized checklists**: Ensuring all discharge elements are addressed

- **Patient engagement**: Active participation in discharge planning decisions

Medication Optimization Program:

- **Pharmacist consultation**: Clinical pharmacist reviews all discharge medications

- **Patient education**: Standardized teaching using teach-back method

- **Medication packaging**: Pill organizers and simplified packaging provided

- **Community pharmacy coordination**: Direct communication about medication changes

Transition Support Services:

- **Bridge clinic**: Same-day or next-day appointments with hospital-based providers

- **Peer support**: Trained peer specialists contact patients within 48 hours

- **Care coordination**: Dedicated staff ensure smooth handoffs to community providers

- **Transportation assistance**: Vouchers and coordination for follow-up appointments

Family Engagement Enhancement:

- **Family meetings**: Structured sessions involving patients, families, and treatment team

- **Educational materials**: Written and video resources about mental illness and recovery

- **Support group referrals**: Connections to ongoing family support programs

- **Crisis planning**: Collaborative development of crisis prevention and response plans

Outcome Measurement and Monitoring:

Process Measures:

- **Discharge planning timeliness**: Percentage of patients with day-one planning initiation

- **Medication education completion**: Documentation of teach-back method use

- **Follow-up appointment scheduling**: Percentage of patients with confirmed appointments

- **Family engagement**: Participation rates in discharge planning meetings

Outcome Measures:

- **30-day readmission rates**: Primary outcome tracked monthly

- **Follow-up appointment attendance**: Percentage attending first outpatient appointment

- **Patient satisfaction**: Scores related to discharge planning and preparation

- **Length of stay**: Average days from admission to discharge

Balancing Measures:

- **Staff satisfaction**: Workload perception and job satisfaction scores

- **Cost analysis**: Total cost per patient including readmission costs

- **Safety incidents**: Medication errors and other adverse events

- **Emergency department visits**: Use of ED services by discharged patients

Six-Month Results: The QI project demonstrates significant improvements across multiple measures:

Primary Outcomes:

- **Readmission rate**: Decreased from 28% to 16% (exceeded goal of 18%)

- **Follow-up attendance**: Increased from 60% to 84% (exceeded goal of 80%)

- **Patient satisfaction**: Improved from 3.2 to 4.3 (exceeded goal of 4.0)

- **Planning timeliness**: 95% of patients have discharge planning initiated within 24 hours

Secondary Benefits:

- **Staff satisfaction**: Improved due to better organization and clearer processes

- **Cost savings**: Reduced readmissions save hospital $450,000 annually

- **Community relationships**: Stronger partnerships with outpatient providers

- **Regulatory compliance**: Improved performance on quality metrics

QI Case Study 14.2: Improving Staff Competence in Suicide Risk Assessment

The psychiatric emergency department identifies concerning patterns in suicide risk assessment documentation: 30% of assessments lack required elements, staff confidence in risk evaluation varies widely, and two sentinel events occurred involving patients whose risk was underestimated. The nursing leadership team launches a comprehensive competency improvement project.

Current State Assessment:

Competency Evaluation: The team conducts systematic assessment of current suicide risk assessment practices:

Documentation Review:

- **Chart audit**: Random review of 100 suicide risk assessments from past six months

- **Missing elements**: Identified gaps in assessment documentation

- **Inconsistency patterns**: Variations in assessment quality between nurses

- **Risk stratification**: Accuracy of risk level assignments compared to outcomes

Staff Self-Assessment:

- **Confidence surveys**: Nurses rate their comfort with suicide risk assessment

- **Knowledge testing**: Formal evaluation of suicide risk factor knowledge

- **Experience inventory**: Documentation of training and clinical experience

- **Learning needs**: Self-identified areas for improvement

Simulation Testing:

- **Standardized scenarios**: All nurses complete suicide risk assessment simulations

- **Skill demonstration**: Observation of assessment techniques and communication

- **Decision-making**: Evaluation of risk stratification and safety planning

- **Documentation**: Review of assessment documentation in simulated cases

Evidence-Based Competency Framework Development:

Literature Review Findings: Research identifies key components of effective suicide risk assessment training:

Assessment Skills:

- **Risk factor identification**: Systematic evaluation of static and dynamic risk factors

- **Protective factor assessment**: Recognition of factors that reduce suicide risk

- **Communication techniques**: Effective questioning about suicidal thoughts and plans

- **Documentation standards**: Comprehensive and accurate record-keeping

Decision-Making Competencies:

- **Risk stratification**: Appropriate assignment of low, moderate, or high-risk levels

- **Safety planning**: Collaborative development of crisis intervention strategies

- **Intervention selection**: Choosing appropriate immediate and long-term interventions

- **Consultation utilization**: Knowing when to seek additional expertise

Training Program Design: The team develops comprehensive competency-based training program:

Educational Components:

- **Online modules**: Self-paced learning about suicide risk factors and assessment tools

- **Classroom sessions**: Interactive workshops with case discussions

- **Simulation practice**: Hands-on experience with standardized patients

- **Mentorship program**: Pairing experienced nurses with those developing skills

Assessment Methods:

- **Written examinations**: Testing knowledge of risk factors and assessment principles

- **Simulation evaluation**: Observed performance in standardized scenarios

- **Portfolio development**: Collection of assessed cases with supervisor feedback

- **Peer review**: Colleague observation and feedback on assessment skills

Implementation Strategy:

Phased Rollout: The training program launches in phases to ensure quality and manageability:

Phase 1: Experienced nurses complete advanced training and become mentors **Phase 2**: All nursing staff complete basic competency requirements **Phase 3**: Ongoing maintenance training and annual competency validation **Phase 4**: Integration into orientation program for new staff

Support Systems:

- **Clinical decision support**: Electronic tools embedded in documentation systems

- **Consultation services**: 24/7 access to psychiatric nurses with specialized expertise

- **Peer support**: Regular case review meetings for difficult assessments

- **Quality feedback**: Individual feedback on assessment accuracy and documentation

Outcome Measurement:

Competency Metrics:

- **Training completion**: Percentage of staff completing required training modules

- **Simulation scores**: Performance ratings on standardized assessment scenarios

- **Knowledge retention**: Scores on periodic knowledge assessments

- **Confidence levels**: Self-reported comfort with suicide risk assessment

Clinical Outcomes:

- **Documentation quality**: Improvement in assessment completeness and accuracy

- **Risk stratification accuracy**: Correlation between assessed risk and actual outcomes

- **Safety plan development**: Quality and completeness of crisis intervention plans

- **Sentinel events**: Reduction in adverse outcomes related to suicide risk assessment

Six-Month Results: The competency improvement project achieves significant improvements:

Training Outcomes:

- **Completion rate**: 98% of staff complete required training within timeline

- **Knowledge scores**: Average improvement of 25% on post-training assessments

- **Simulation performance**: 90% of nurses demonstrate competent assessment skills

- **Confidence levels**: Significant improvement in self-reported competence

Clinical Improvements:

- **Documentation quality**: 95% of assessments include all required elements (up from 70%)

- **Risk accuracy**: Improved correlation between assessed risk and clinical outcomes

- **Safety planning**: 100% of high-risk patients have documented safety plans

- **Adverse events**: No sentinel events related to suicide risk assessment in six months

Research Translation and Evidence Implementation

Effective quality improvement requires systematic approaches to identifying, evaluating, and implementing new evidence in clinical practice. This process transforms research findings into improved patient care while ensuring changes are sustainable and effective.

QI Case Study 14.3: Implementing Trauma-Informed Care

The community mental health center serves a population with high rates of trauma exposure, but staff lack systematic training in trauma-informed care principles. Research demonstrates that trauma-informed approaches improve engagement, reduce re-traumatization, and enhance treatment outcomes. The center launches a comprehensive implementation project.

Evidence Review and Adaptation:

Literature Search Strategy: The implementation team conducts systematic review of trauma-informed care evidence:

Database Searches:

- **PubMed**: Medical and nursing literature

- **PsycINFO**: Psychology and mental health research

- **CINAHL**: Nursing and allied health databases

- **Cochrane**: Systematic reviews and meta-analyses

Evidence Quality Assessment:

- **Study design**: Preference for randomized controlled trials and systematic reviews

- **Population relevance**: Studies involving similar patient populations

- **Outcome measures**: Research addressing engagement, satisfaction, and clinical outcomes

- **Implementation factors**: Studies describing successful implementation strategies

Key Findings:

- **Engagement improvement**: Trauma-informed approaches increase treatment retention by 20-30%

- **Symptom reduction**: Enhanced outcomes for PTSD, depression, and anxiety

- **Staff satisfaction**: Improved job satisfaction and reduced burnout

- **Cost effectiveness**: Reduced treatment dropout and improved resource utilization

Adaptation for Local Context: The team adapts evidence-based trauma-informed care principles for their specific setting:

Population Characteristics:

- **Demographics**: Primarily low-income, diverse ethnic communities

- **Trauma types**: High rates of childhood abuse, domestic violence, and community violence

- **Service utilization**: Frequent treatment dropout and crisis service use

- **Cultural factors**: Multiple languages and cultural backgrounds represented

Organizational Assessment:

- **Current practices**: Limited trauma screening and trauma-specific treatments

- **Staff readiness**: Mixed levels of trauma knowledge and comfort

- **Resource availability**: Funding constraints and staffing limitations

- **Leadership support**: Strong commitment from administration

Implementation Planning:

Stakeholder Engagement: Successful implementation requires buy-in from multiple stakeholder groups:

Staff Preparation:

- **Education sessions**: Training on trauma prevalence, impact, and recovery principles

- **Skill development**: Communication techniques and trauma-sensitive interventions

- **Self-care training**: Recognizing and managing secondary trauma exposure

- **Culture change**: Shifting from "What's wrong with you?" to "What happened to you?"

Patient and Family Engagement:

- **Education materials**: Information about trauma and recovery in multiple languages

- **Choice enhancement**: Increased options and control in treatment planning

- **Safety emphasis**: Creating emotionally and physically safe environments

- **Strength focus**: Recognizing resilience and survival skills

System Changes:

- **Screening protocols**: Universal trauma screening for all new patients

- **Environmental modifications**: Creating welcoming, non-threatening spaces

- **Policy updates**: Revising policies to reflect trauma-informed principles

- **Staff support**: Employee assistance programs and peer support systems

Training Curriculum Development: The team develops comprehensive training program based on evidence and organizational needs:

Core Competencies:

- **Trauma knowledge**: Understanding prevalence, types, and impacts of trauma

- **Assessment skills**: Trauma screening and evaluation techniques

- **Intervention approaches**: Trauma-specific and trauma-informed treatments

- **Self-care practices**: Managing secondary trauma and maintaining professional wellbeing

Training Methods:

- **Didactic sessions**: Classroom instruction on trauma theory and evidence

- **Interactive workshops**: Skill practice and case study discussions

- **Simulation exercises**: Practice with standardized patients

- **Peer consultation**: Regular case review and mutual support

Sustainability Planning:

- **Train-the-trainer**: Developing internal capacity for ongoing education

- **Integration**: Incorporating trauma-informed principles into all policies and procedures

- **Continuous learning**: Regular updates and refresher training

- **Quality monitoring**: Ongoing assessment of implementation fidelity

Outcome Measurement Framework:

Implementation Metrics:

- **Training completion**: Percentage of staff completing required education

- **Knowledge assessment**: Pre- and post-training test scores

- **Screening rates**: Percentage of patients receiving trauma screening

- **Documentation quality**: Completeness of trauma-related assessment and planning

Clinical Outcomes:

- **Engagement**: Treatment retention and appointment attendance rates

- **Satisfaction**: Patient and family satisfaction with services

- **Symptom improvement**: Standardized outcome measures for trauma symptoms

- **Crisis utilization**: Emergency department visits and crisis interventions

Staff Outcomes:

- **Job satisfaction**: Staff satisfaction surveys and turnover rates

- **Burnout measures**: Professional quality of life assessments

- **Competence**: Self-reported confidence in trauma-informed care

- **Culture assessment**: Organizational climate and culture surveys

Twelve-Month Results: The trauma-informed care implementation demonstrates significant positive impacts:

Implementation Success:

- **Training completion**: 96% of staff complete required trauma-informed care training

- **Screening implementation**: 88% of new patients receive trauma screening

- **Documentation improvement**: Significant increase in trauma-related assessment documentation

- **Policy integration**: All major policies revised to reflect trauma-informed principles

Clinical Improvements:

- **Treatment retention**: 25% increase in completion of recommended treatment episodes

- **Patient satisfaction**: Significant improvement in satisfaction with services

- **Symptom outcomes**: Enhanced improvements in PTSD and depression measures

- **Crisis reduction**: 20% decrease in emergency department visits by regular patients

Staff Benefits:

- **Job satisfaction**: Improved satisfaction scores and reduced turnover

- **Competence**: Increased confidence in working with trauma survivors

- **Secondary trauma**: Reduced burnout and secondary trauma symptoms

- **Culture change**: More supportive and collaborative work environment

Building Quality Improvement Competence

Quality improvement represents a fundamental competency for all psychiatric nurses. Your ability to identify problems, search for evidence, implement changes, and measure outcomes determines your effectiveness as a clinician and your contribution to the profession's advancement.

Successful QI work requires both technical skills (data analysis, project management, outcome measurement) and interpersonal skills (stakeholder engagement, change management, team leadership). These competencies develop through education, practice, and mentorship from experienced QI practitioners.

The next chapter examines how professional development and self-care practices support your ability to provide excellent patient care while maintaining your own wellbeing throughout your nursing career.

Quality Improvement Foundations

- Systematic problem identification and root cause analysis guide effective QI project development

- Evidence-based interventions provide the foundation for quality improvement initiatives

- Stakeholder engagement and change management are essential for successful implementation

- Outcome measurement must include process measures, clinical outcomes, and balancing measures

- Research translation requires systematic approaches to evaluating and adapting evidence for local contexts

- Sustainability planning ensures that improvements continue beyond initial implementation phases

- Staff competency development improves both clinical outcomes and professional satisfaction

- Quality improvement skills are fundamental competencies for all psychiatric nurses

Chapter 15: Professional Development and Self-Care

The alarm goes off at 5:30 AM for another twelve-hour shift in the psychiatric intensive care unit. As you pour your coffee, you reflect on yesterday's challenges: a young patient's first psychotic break, a colleague's resignation due to burnout, and your own growing sense that you need something more from your nursing career. Professional development and self-care aren't luxuries in psychiatric nursing—they're necessities for maintaining both the quality of care you provide and your own wellbeing over the course of your career.

Your professional journey in psychiatric nursing extends far beyond acquiring initial competencies. The field continues to change with new treatments, evolving patient populations, and emerging challenges that require ongoing learning and adaptation. Equally important is developing the resilience and self-awareness needed to sustain yourself through the emotional demands of caring for people in psychological distress.

Resilience Building Through Evidence-Based Strategies

Resilience—the ability to adapt and thrive despite adversity—represents a learnable set of skills rather than an innate personality trait. Research identifies specific strategies that help healthcare workers maintain effectiveness and wellbeing even under challenging circumstances.

Professional Development Case Study 15.1: Building Resilience After Traumatic Patient Death

Sarah, a psychiatric nurse with five years of experience, struggles with intense grief and self-doubt following the suicide death of a long-term patient she had worked with for eight months. Despite following all protocols and providing excellent care, she blames herself for not preventing the tragedy and considers leaving psychiatric nursing entirely.

Understanding Resilience Factors:

Research-Based Resilience Components: Evidence identifies multiple factors that contribute to professional resilience:

Cognitive Flexibility:

- **Perspective-taking**: Ability to view situations from multiple angles
- **Realistic thinking**: Balancing optimism with accurate assessment of challenges
- **Growth mindset**: Viewing difficulties as opportunities for learning and development

- **Self-compassion**: Treating oneself with kindness during difficult times

Emotional Regulation:

- **Stress management**: Effective techniques for managing acute and chronic stress
- **Emotional awareness**: Recognition and understanding of one's emotional responses
- **Coping strategies**: Healthy approaches to managing difficult emotions
- **Support utilization**: Willingness to seek and accept help from others

Professional Identity:

- **Purpose clarity**: Clear understanding of professional values and goals
- **Competence confidence**: Realistic assessment of skills and abilities
- **Professional boundaries**: Appropriate limits on emotional involvement
- **Meaning-making**: Finding significance and value in nursing work

Social Connection:

- **Peer support**: Relationships with colleagues who understand professional challenges
- **Mentorship**: Guidance from experienced nurses and other professionals
- **Professional community**: Involvement in nursing organizations and professional activities
- **Personal relationships**: Strong connections outside of work environment

Resilience Assessment and Planning:

Sarah's Resilience Evaluation: A systematic assessment reveals Sarah's current resilience strengths and areas for development:

Strengths Identified:

- **Clinical competence**: Excellent nursing skills and patient rapport
- **Professional commitment**: Strong dedication to psychiatric nursing
- **Empathy**: Deep caring for patients and their wellbeing
- **Learning orientation**: Willingness to seek feedback and improve practice

Areas for Development:

- **Self-blame patterns**: Tendency to take excessive responsibility for patient outcomes
- **Perfectionist thinking**: Unrealistic expectations for preventing all negative outcomes
- **Isolation behavior**: Withdrawing from colleagues when experiencing distress
- **Limited coping strategies**: Over-reliance on work as primary source of meaning

Individualized Resilience Plan: Sarah works with a mentor to develop a personalized resilience-building strategy:

Cognitive Skill Development:

- **Realistic thinking practice**: Learning to evaluate situations objectively
- **Self-compassion exercises**: Treating herself with same kindness she shows patients
- **Professional responsibility clarification**: Understanding limits of nursing influence
- **Growth mindset cultivation**: Viewing challenges as learning opportunities

Emotional Regulation Training:

- **Mindfulness meditation**: Daily practice for stress reduction and emotional awareness
- **Journaling**: Written reflection on experiences and emotions
- **Physical exercise**: Regular activity for stress management and mood improvement
- **Professional counseling**: Individual therapy to process grief and trauma

Professional Community Engagement:

- **Peer support group**: Participation in hospital-based nurse support group
- **Mentorship relationship**: Regular meetings with experienced psychiatric nurse
- **Professional development**: Attendance at conferences and continuing education
- **Volunteer activities**: Contributing to nursing profession through committee work

Personal Life Enhancement:

- **Hobby development**: Pursuing interests outside of nursing

- **Relationship strengthening**: Investing time in family and friendships

- **Spiritual practices**: Exploring sources of meaning and purpose

- **Work-life boundaries**: Establishing clear limits on work-related activities

Six-Month Outcomes: Sarah demonstrates significant improvement in resilience and professional satisfaction:

Personal Growth:

- **Self-compassion**: Reduced self-blame and increased kindness toward herself

- **Emotional regulation**: Better management of work-related stress and grief

- **Perspective**: More realistic understanding of professional responsibilities

- **Coping skills**: Diverse strategies for managing difficult situations

Professional Development:

- **Clinical confidence**: Renewed sense of competence and effectiveness

- **Peer relationships**: Stronger connections with colleagues

- **Career commitment**: Renewed dedication to psychiatric nursing

- **Leadership emergence**: Beginning to mentor newer nurses

Secondary Trauma Prevention and Management

Healthcare workers, particularly those in psychiatric settings, face significant risk for secondary trauma—psychological distress resulting from exposure to others' traumatic experiences. Understanding and preventing secondary trauma is essential for career sustainability.

Professional Development Case Study 15.2: Managing Secondary Trauma in Emergency Psychiatry

Michael, an emergency psychiatric nurse with three years of experience, begins experiencing symptoms that mirror those of his patients: intrusive thoughts about violent incidents he's witnessed, hypervigilance during his commute home, and emotional numbing in his personal relationships. He recognizes these as signs of secondary trauma but isn't sure how to address them.

Secondary Trauma Recognition:

Symptom Identification: Secondary trauma can manifest in various ways:

Cognitive Symptoms:

- **Intrusive thoughts**: Recurring images or memories of patient trauma stories
- **Difficulty concentrating**: Problems focusing on tasks at work and home
- **Cynicism**: Increasingly negative worldview and loss of hope
- **Memory problems**: Difficulty remembering details or feeling mentally foggy

Emotional Symptoms:

- **Emotional numbing**: Reduced ability to feel positive emotions
- **Increased anxiety**: Heightened worry about safety and danger
- **Depression**: Persistent sadness and loss of interest in activities
- **Irritability**: Increased anger and reduced patience with others

Physical Symptoms:

- **Sleep disturbances**: Difficulty falling asleep or staying asleep
- **Fatigue**: Persistent tiredness despite adequate rest
- **Headaches**: Frequent tension headaches or migraines
- **Gastrointestinal issues**: Stomach problems, appetite changes

Behavioral Changes:

- **Avoidance**: Staying away from certain patients or situations
- **Social withdrawal**: Reduced engagement with family and friends
- **Substance use**: Increased alcohol or drug use for coping
- **Work performance**: Decreased effectiveness or increased absences

Risk Factor Assessment: Certain factors increase vulnerability to secondary trauma:

Individual Risk Factors:

- **Personal trauma history**: Previous traumatic experiences increase susceptibility

- **High empathy**: Strong emotional connection to patient suffering

- **Limited experience**: Newer nurses may lack developed coping strategies

- **Perfectionist tendencies**: Unrealistic expectations for helping all patients

Workplace Risk Factors:

- **High trauma exposure**: Frequent contact with severely traumatized patients

- **Limited support**: Inadequate supervision or peer support systems

- **Workload pressure**: High patient-to-nurse ratios and time constraints

- **Organizational culture**: Lack of trauma awareness or support resources

Prevention Strategies Implementation:

Individual Prevention Approaches: Michael implements evidence-based strategies for preventing and managing secondary trauma:

Awareness and Education:

- **Symptom recognition**: Learning to identify early signs of secondary trauma

- **Trauma understanding**: Education about normal responses to trauma exposure

- **Risk factor awareness**: Understanding personal and workplace vulnerabilities

- **Resource identification**: Knowing available support services and interventions

Self-Care Practices:

- **Physical self-care**: Regular exercise, adequate sleep, and healthy nutrition

- **Emotional self-care**: Mindfulness, relaxation techniques, and emotional expression

- **Social self-care**: Maintaining relationships and seeking support from others

- **Spiritual self-care**: Engaging in activities that provide meaning and purpose

Professional Boundaries:

- **Emotional boundaries**: Maintaining appropriate emotional distance from patient trauma

- **Time boundaries**: Limiting work hours and taking regular breaks

- **Role boundaries**: Understanding professional responsibilities and limitations
- **Information boundaries**: Avoiding excessive exposure to traumatic details

Organizational Prevention Strategies: The emergency department implements systematic approaches to reduce secondary trauma risk:

Staff Support Programs:

- **Employee assistance**: Confidential counseling and support services
- **Peer support teams**: Trained colleagues providing mutual support
- **Critical incident debriefing**: Structured processing after difficult cases
- **Wellness committees**: Groups focused on staff wellbeing and support

Training and Education:

- **Secondary trauma education**: Training on recognition and prevention
- **Stress management**: Workshops on coping strategies and resilience building
- **Communication skills**: Training in difficult conversations and conflict resolution
- **Self-care planning**: Helping staff develop personalized wellness strategies

Environmental Modifications:

- **Workload management**: Ensuring reasonable patient assignments and break time
- **Physical environment**: Creating calm, supportive spaces for staff
- **Schedule flexibility**: Allowing time off for recovery after difficult cases
- **Resource availability**: Providing access to support materials and services

Professional Counseling and Support: Michael engages with professional counseling to address secondary trauma symptoms:

Trauma-Focused Therapy:

- **Cognitive processing**: Working through traumatic images and thoughts
- **Emotional regulation**: Learning skills for managing intense emotions
- **Meaning-making**: Finding purpose and growth through difficult experiences

- **Coping skill development**: Building healthy strategies for ongoing stress management

Group Support:

- **Peer support groups**: Meeting with other healthcare workers experiencing similar challenges

- **Professional discussion**: Processing difficult cases with colleagues

- **Family education**: Helping family understand secondary trauma impacts

- **Community resources**: Connecting with broader support networks

Career Pathways in Psychiatric Nursing

Psychiatric nursing offers diverse career opportunities that allow for professional growth, specialization, and leadership development. Understanding available pathways helps you make informed decisions about your professional development.

Professional Development Case Study 15.3: Advanced Practice Career Development

Jennifer, a staff nurse with seven years of psychiatric nursing experience, feels ready for new challenges and increased autonomy in her practice. She's considering returning to school for advanced practice credentials but wants to understand her options and develop a realistic career plan.

Advanced Practice Roles in Psychiatric Nursing (35, 36, 37):

Psychiatric-Mental Health Nurse Practitioner (PMHNP): PMHNPs provide comprehensive psychiatric care across the lifespan:

Scope of Practice:

- **Assessment and diagnosis**: Comprehensive psychiatric evaluations

- **Medication management**: Prescribing and monitoring psychiatric medications

- **Psychotherapy**: Individual, group, and family therapy

- **Consultation**: Collaborating with other healthcare providers

Educational Requirements:

- **Master's or doctoral degree**: Graduate education in psychiatric-mental health nursing

- **Clinical hours**: Supervised practice in various psychiatric settings

- **National certification**: Examination through American Nurses Credentialing Center

- **State licensing**: Meeting individual state requirements for advanced practice

Practice Settings:

- **Outpatient clinics**: Community mental health centers and private practice

- **Hospital consultation**: Liaison psychiatry and consultation services

- **Primary care integration**: Embedded mental health services

- **Specialty programs**: Addiction treatment, forensic psychiatry, geriatric psychiatry

Clinical Nurse Specialist (CNS): Psychiatric CNS roles focus on improving patient outcomes and nursing practice:

Core Functions:

- **Direct patient care**: Expert clinical practice with complex patients

- **Consultation**: Advising nurses and other professionals about psychiatric care

- **Education**: Teaching nurses, patients, and families

- **Research**: Conducting and implementing evidence-based practice

Specialization Areas:

- **Population focus**: Child and adolescent, adult, or geriatric psychiatry

- **Setting specialization**: Inpatient units, emergency services, or community programs

- **Condition expertise**: Mood disorders, psychosis, addiction, or trauma

- **Quality improvement**: Leading initiatives to improve care quality

Nurse Administrator and Leadership Roles: Leadership positions allow nurses to influence psychiatric care delivery:

Management Positions:

- **Unit managers**: Overseeing day-to-day operations of psychiatric units

- **Program directors**: Leading specialized programs or services

- **Department directors**: Managing entire psychiatric nursing departments
- **Chief nursing officers**: Executive leadership in psychiatric facilities

Policy and Advocacy Roles:

- **Quality improvement**: Leading organizational change initiatives
- **Policy development**: Creating and implementing clinical policies
- **Professional advocacy**: Representing nursing interests in healthcare policy
- **Community leadership**: Participating in community mental health planning

Education and Training Roles: Teaching positions contribute to the development of future psychiatric nurses:

Academic Positions:

- **Faculty roles**: Teaching in nursing schools and universities
- **Clinical instructors**: Supervising students in clinical settings
- **Continuing education**: Providing ongoing education for practicing nurses
- **Simulation specialists**: Developing and implementing simulation-based training

Clinical Education:

- **Staff development**: Coordinating education for nursing staff
- **Orientation programs**: Training new nurses in psychiatric nursing
- **Specialty training**: Developing expertise in specific areas
- **Mentorship coordination**: Facilitating mentoring relationships

Research and Scholarship Opportunities: Research roles advance the scientific foundation of psychiatric nursing:

Clinical Research:

- **Intervention studies**: Testing new approaches to psychiatric nursing care
- **Outcomes research**: Evaluating effectiveness of nursing interventions
- **Quality improvement**: Studying methods for improving care delivery

- **Health services research**: Examining healthcare delivery systems

Academic Research:

- **Faculty positions**: Conducting research in university settings

- **Grant writing**: Securing funding for nursing research projects

- **Publication**: Contributing to professional literature

- **Conference presentations**: Sharing research findings with professional communities

Career Planning and Development Strategy:

Self-Assessment and Goal Setting: Jennifer completes comprehensive self-assessment to guide career planning:

Strengths and Interests Evaluation:

- **Clinical skills**: Assessment of current competencies and areas for growth

- **Interest areas**: Identification of preferred patient populations and settings

- **Values clarification**: Understanding what matters most in professional work

- **Lifestyle considerations**: Balancing career goals with personal priorities

Career Goal Development:

- **Short-term goals** (1-2 years): Continuing education and skill development

- **Medium-term goals** (3-5 years): Graduate education and certification

- **Long-term goals** (5-10 years): Advanced practice role establishment

- **Ultimate aspirations**: Leadership positions and professional contributions

Educational Planning: Jennifer researches graduate programs and develops education plan:

Program Selection Criteria:

- **Accreditation**: Ensuring programs meet professional standards

- **Faculty expertise**: Finding programs with strong psychiatric nursing faculty

- **Clinical experiences**: Availability of diverse psychiatric practice opportunities

- **Flexibility**: Options for part-time study or online components

- **Financial considerations**: Tuition costs and financial aid availability

Preparation Activities:

- **Prerequisites**: Completing any required undergraduate courses

- **GRE preparation**: Test preparation if required for admission

- **Application development**: Personal statements and recommendation letters

- **Financial planning**: Exploring funding options and budget planning

Professional Development Activities: While preparing for graduate school, Jennifer engages in professional development:

Continuing Education:

- **Conference attendance**: Psychiatric nursing conferences and workshops

- **Specialty training**: Certification programs in specific areas of interest

- **Online learning**: Web-based courses and professional development modules

- **Reading**: Professional journals and current literature

Professional Involvement:

- **Association membership**: Joining American Psychiatric Nurses Association (38)

- **Committee participation**: Volunteering for professional committees

- **Networking**: Building relationships with advanced practice nurses

- **Mentorship**: Finding mentors in desired career areas

Certification Preparation and Maintenance:

ANCC PMH-BC Certification (39, 40): The American Nurses Credentialing Center offers certification for psychiatric-mental health nurses:

Eligibility Requirements:

- **Education**: Bachelor's degree in nursing from accredited program

- **Practice hours**: 2,000 hours of psychiatric nursing practice within three years

- **Continuing education**: 30 hours of psychiatric nursing education

- **Professional development**: Evidence of ongoing learning and competence

Examination Preparation:

- **Content areas**: Psychopathology, therapeutic relationships, psychopharmacology, milieu management

- **Study resources**: Review courses, textbooks, and practice examinations

- **Study groups**: Collaborative preparation with other nurses

- **Practice tests**: Familiarization with examination format and content

Certification Maintenance:

- **Continuing education**: 75 hours every five years

- **Practice requirements**: Ongoing psychiatric nursing practice

- **Professional activities**: Contributions to psychiatric nursing profession

- **Recertification**: Meeting renewal requirements and fee payment

Building a Sustainable Career

Long-term success in psychiatric nursing requires intentional career management that balances professional growth with personal wellbeing. This includes developing expertise, building professional networks, and maintaining the resilience needed for sustained practice.

Professional Portfolio Development: Document your achievements, skills, and contributions to demonstrate professional growth:

- **Clinical accomplishments**: Certifications, training, and special skills

- **Educational achievements**: Degrees, continuing education, and presentations

- **Professional contributions**: Committee work, publications, and volunteer activities

- **Quality improvement**: Projects and initiatives you've led or participated in

Networking and Mentorship: Build relationships that support your professional development:

- **Peer networks**: Colleagues who share similar interests and challenges

- **Mentorship relationships**: Both serving as mentee and mentor to others

- **Professional associations**: Active participation in nursing organizations

- **Interprofessional connections**: Relationships with other healthcare professionals

Work-Life Integration: Maintain balance between professional demands and personal life:

- **Boundary setting**: Clear limits on work hours and availability

- **Self-care practices**: Regular activities that support physical and emotional health

- **Relationship maintenance**: Investing time in family and friendships

- **Personal interests**: Hobbies and activities unrelated to nursing work

Closing Wisdom

Your career in psychiatric nursing represents more than a job—it's a calling that offers opportunities to make profound differences in people's lives while contributing to your own growth and development. The patients you serve will teach you about resilience, courage, and human dignity in ways that textbooks cannot capture.

Professional development and self-care aren't optional extras in psychiatric nursing—they're essential elements that determine both your effectiveness as a clinician and your satisfaction as a person. The time and energy you invest in building resilience, preventing secondary trauma, and planning your career will return to you many times over in terms of job satisfaction, clinical competence, and personal fulfillment.

The psychiatric nursing profession needs nurses like you who are committed to excellence, continuous learning, and compassionate care. Your willingness to grow professionally while caring for yourself personally ensures that you'll be available to serve patients throughout a long and meaningful career.

Professional Excellence Foundations

- Resilience can be developed through evidence-based strategies including cognitive flexibility, emotional regulation, and social connection

- Secondary trauma prevention requires both individual self-care practices and organizational support systems

- Career pathways in psychiatric nursing offer diverse opportunities for specialization and leadership development

- Professional development planning should include self-assessment, goal setting, and systematic skill building

- Certification and continuing education demonstrate commitment to professional excellence

- Sustainable careers require balance between professional growth and personal wellbeing

- Mentorship relationships benefit both mentors and mentees in professional development

- Self-care practices are essential for maintaining effectiveness and preventing burnout

References

(1) The Revised AACN Essentials: Implications for Nursing Regulation. Journal of Nursing Regulation. 2022.

(2) AACN Essentials as the Conceptual Thread of Nursing Education. PubMed. 2022.

(3) Case Study Method and Problem-Based Learning: Utilizing the Pedagogical Model of Progressive Complexity in Nursing Education. De Gruyter. 2011.

(4) Effects of an unfolding case study on clinical reasoning, self-directed learning, and team collaboration of undergraduate nursing students: A mixed methods study. ScienceDirect. 2024.

(5) Depressed and Suicidal Patients in the Emergency Department: An Evidence-Based Approach. EB Medicine. 2023.

(6) Validated Screening Tools. VA MIRECC. 2023.

(7) A validation study of PHQ-9 suicide item with the Columbia Suicide Severity Rating Scale in outpatients with mood disorders at National Network of Depression Centers. ScienceDirect. 2022.

(8) The PHQ-9 Item 9 based screening for suicide risk: a validation study of the Patient Health Questionnaire (PHQ)-9 Item 9 with the Columbia Suicide Severity Rating Scale (C-SSRS). ScienceDirect. 2018.

(9) Tools for Cognitive Screening & Assessment in Nursing Home Residents (Part 2). GuideStar Eldercare. 2023.

(10) Montreal Cognitive Assessment (MoCA). MoCA Cognition. 2023.

(11) The DSM-5 Cultural Formulation Interview and the Evolution of Cultural Assessment in Psychiatry. Psychiatric Times. 2020.

(12) An Introduction to the Cultural Formulation Interview. Psychiatry Online. 2020.

(13) Our Standards for Behavioral Health Accreditation. The Joint Commission. 2023.

(14) Joint Commission Rights Standards: New Requirements. Barrins & Associates. 2023.

(15) Relationship between nurses' use of verbal de-escalation and mechanical restraint in acute inpatient mental health care: a retrospective study. Wiley Online Library. 2022.

(16) De-escalating aggression in acute inpatient mental health settings: a behaviour change theory-informed, secondary qualitative analysis of staff and patient perspectives. BMC Psychiatry. 2024.

(17) Trauma-Informed Nursing Practice. OJIN: The Online Journal of Issues in Nursing. 2019.

(18) The State of Telehealth Before and After the COVID-19 Pandemic. PubMed Central. 2022.

(19) Impact of the COVID-19 Pandemic on the Global Delivery of Mental Health Services and Telemental Health: Systematic Review. JMIR Mental Health. 2022.

(20) Training of NANDA-I Nursing Diagnoses (NDs), Nursing Interventions Classification (NIC) and Nursing Outcomes Classification (NOC), in Psychiatric Wards: A randomized controlled trial. ResearchGate. 2019.

(21) Training of NANDA-I Nursing Diagnoses (NDs), Nursing Interventions Classification (NIC) and Nursing Outcomes Classification (NOC), in Psychiatric Wards: A randomized controlled trial. PMC. 2019.

(22) Electronic nursing care plans through the use of NANDA, NOC, and NIC taxonomies in community setting: A descriptive study in northern Italy. PubMed Central. 2022.

(23) NANDA-I, NIC, and NOC taxonomies, patients' satisfaction, and nurses' perception of the work environment: an Italian cross-sectional pilot study. ResearchGate. 2020.

(24) Training of NANDA-I Nursing Diagnoses (NDs), Nursing Interventions Classification (NIC) and Nursing Outcomes Classification (NOC), in Psychiatric Wards: A randomized controlled trial. ResearchGate. 2019.

(25) The State of Telehealth Before and After the COVID-19 Pandemic. PubMed Central. 2022.

(26) Impact of the COVID-19 Pandemic on the Global Delivery of Mental Health Services and Telemental Health: Systematic Review. JMIR Mental Health. 2022.

(27) Peer Support Workers for those in Recovery. SAMHSA. 2023.

(28) Peer Support in Mental Health: Literature Review. PubMed Central. 2020.

(29) CMS Psychotherapy Documentation Requirements: Complete Guide. Mentalyc. 2023.

(30) Inpatient Psychiatric Services. Centers for Medicare & Medicaid Services. 2023.

(31) Climate Change and Mental Health Connections. American Psychiatric Association. 2023.

(32) The relationship between climate change and mental health: a systematic review of the association between eco-anxiety, psychological distress, and symptoms of major affective disorders. BMC Psychiatry. 2024.

(33) A Path to Improved Health Care Worker Well-Being: Lessons from the COVID-19 Pandemic. National Academy of Medicine. 2021.

(34) A rapid review of the impact of COVID-19 on the mental health of healthcare workers: implications for supporting psychological well-being. BMC Public Health. 2020.

(35) APNA Position: Psychotherapy and the Scope of the Psychiatric-Mental Health Advanced Practice Registered Nurse Role. American Psychiatric Nurses Association. 2023.

(36) About Psychiatric Advanced Practice Nurses. American Psychiatric Nurses Association. 2023.

(37) Questions about Advanced Practice Psychiatric Nurses. American Psychiatric Nurses Association. 2023.

(38) APNA Position: Diversity, Equity, and Inclusion. American Psychiatric Nurses Association. 2023.

(39) Psychiatric-Mental Health Nurse Practitioner (Across the Lifespan) Certification (PMHNP-BC). American Nurses Credentialing Center. 2023.

(40) Psychiatric-Mental Health Nursing Certification (PMH-BC™). American Nurses Credentialing Center. 2023.

www.ingramcontent.com/pod-product-compliance
Lightning Source LLC
Chambersburg PA
CBHW081151270326

41930CB00014B/3112